No Ordinary Joe

Joe de Souza

Published by Joe de Souza, 2023.

While every precaution has been taken in the preparation of this book, the publisher assumes no responsibility for errors or omissions, or for damages resulting from the use of the information contained herein.

NO ORDINARY JOE

First edition. February 1, 2023.

ISBN: 979-8215130650

Written by Joe de Souza.

Table of Contents

Introduction 1

Chapter 1 | Boyhood 4

Chapter 2 | The beginning of illness | and the importance of friends..10

Chapter 3 | My first breakdown 17

Chapter 4 | Edward de Souza...22

Chapter 5 | Longrove and Horton hospitals 26

Chapter 6 | The Escape...31

Chapter 7 | The rabbits and the gun 35

Chapter 8 | The waiting room...36

Chapter 9 | The highs, the lows | and the funny side of grandiosity..39

Chapter 10 | Rupert..44

Chapter 11 | In and out..47

Chapter 12 | Mr 60s...50

Chapter 13 | Plant man 52

Chapter 14 | Pippa 56

Chapter 15 | Ian Powell..60

Chapter 16 | The fishing trip 62

Chapter 17 | Mixed nuts 64

Chapter 18 | We're from the other side...68

Chapter 19 | Bob save the Queen...70

Chapter 20 | The visitor (1990)..72

Chapter 21 | The metal gate, the ring and the funeral | (around 2000 – last hospital stay)...76

Chapter 22 | The stranger 2010..80

Chapter 23 | The river and the unicorn 82

Chapter 24 | The Africa trip...83

Chapter 25 | The spiritual barterer | direct memories of a mad episode...88

Chapter 26 | John Trendy and the Folios Foundation............................89

Chapter 27 | Dan and I take a Christmas trip 93

Chapter 28 | The respect marshal...97

Chapter 29 | Three go mad in Hounslow 99

Chapter 30 | The Cornish sea and the seagull 102

Chapter 31 | Glad you're still with us | (around 1983)................. 104

Chapter 32 | Love, Dan and redemption 107

Chapter 33 | In and out of madness 1980 - 2000 111

Chapter 34 | Daniel.. 115

Conclusion... 118

Epilogue.. 120

Introduction

When I was a child, I had a recurring nightmare. I was at home, surrounded by loved ones, when an overwhelming and overpowering force overtook me. At first, I clung to furniture, to stop the upwards pull. Then I would call my family for help. But the force was too strong, despite their efforts. Soon I was ascending into the sky, so high, that my loved ones became mere specks. Then it would release me, and I would fall back to earth like a lead weight, hitting the ground with a savage thud. Then I awoke.

The dream reflected a future adult life of huge mood swings - highs spiralling out of control followed by plummeting lows. In 1980, when I was eighteen, I began to suffer from severe mental illness. From this point on I was often sectioned and when high, I often escaped. Usually, I would be brought back by the police, over-medicated, and locked in.

I recently estimated the combined total of pills and injections I have had between being eighteen and sixty, and I reckon it's approximately one hundred thousand. But I have lived to tell the tale and I am a proud Dad to a wonderful young man and have not been sectioned or hospitalised since he was born.

This is the story of my experiences of having bipolar with schizo-affective disorder and of all the people I met along the way. It's a sometimes-disjointed story of an illness that has spanned over thirty years of my life, from the first breakdown until now: the years of vulnerability, the huge and out-of-control bipolar highs and the suicidal lows, the sometimes tragic, sometimes humorous accounts of the colourful lives of some of the people I met over that time.

I have attempted suicide often, sometimes with huge overdoses, resulting in unconsciousness. I would come around, attached to a drip and /or a heart monitor and with the prospect of having my stomach pumped. I would then have to take a charcoal-type substance, to soak up the dangerous poisons of the pills. I also attempted to hang myself several times.

As I began to recover, my Mum held my hand like a child and my Dad tried hard to help me walk again. I was often in catatonic depression. 'Come on Joe,' my Dad would say. 'One more step. That's it,' as I would scuff my shoes with each step, like a zombie.

I couldn't read or write. I could barely speak. I shuffled along and wishing to curl up in a foetal position, sleep or die. I took no pleasure from being alive.

It is only through the grace of God, luck, a strong constitution and frankly, my impracticality that I am here today. I simply wasn't very good at killing myself. I have also had a huge amount of support, not only from the care of doctors and nurses but also from close family and friends. My stubborn resistance has helped and, of course, the birth of my son.

I'm more sensible with the life I lead now. I continue to take all the pills and injections that I'm given. The mad and dark thoughts are never far away, but I do know that the medication is keeping me well and out of hospital. When I was manically ill many years ago, there could often be a sense of elation, even euphoria.

'Why,' I would ask, 'is it necessary to lock me away from this lovely, powerful feeling?'

I would look around me at all the sour, bitter faces and think *they're the ones who should be locked up, not me.*

It's a joy that finally, people are beginning to talk about mental illness and discover that it is more common than we once thought. It can be a frightening and lonely experience and can re-emerge and strike at any time. It is also the biggest killer of young men in Britain.

Each story in *No Ordinary Joe* is a separate slice of memory, which exists on its own. However, when put together, you can get to know the characters and build a better picture. If I have succeeded in connecting with anyone who has suffered or who is suffering anything similar and given them hope, then I am delighted.

Chapter 1
Boyhood

Life in our family home was hectic and fun. Never a dull moment. When I was a toddler, we moved from St John's Wood in NW London to Barnes in SW London. Mum told me that I sat on the front step of our old house, crying as the contents of my home were emptied and taken away in a removal van.

I was placed into a local kindergarten, which I can barely remember. Dad told me that once when he came to pick me up, all the children were sitting around in a circle holding hands and I was sitting outside this circle, throwing bits of paper at them.

When settled in, Mum and Dad were busy in their new home and their jobs, as well as looking after three children. When Lu was born, Mum was twenty-four and had three kids under the age of three.

My parents were both actors. At that time, Mum, Miranda Connell, was presenting Play School on the television and Dad was often busy doing radio or a play, and sometimes a film. Once, I looked outside my window to see a huge limousine. He was being whisked off to the South of France to film a clip for an advert for American Express. He looked so small in the back of that huge car.

I never really understood that my parents were famous. It all went over my head, partly because some of my mates also had one or two famous parents and because I grew up with it. I did notice children in school would recognize Mum from presenting Play School, which was a very popular children's television program at the time, but to me, they were just Mum and Dad. Although I do remember that once when Dudley Moore was leaving our house, I didn't know who he was, but I was intrigued by the fact that he was about the same height as my Mum.

Our house was a Mecca for Mum and Dad's friends and their children, and they often held parties. We would misbehave around the house, just as the adults would. Now there were four of us: Tim, me, Lu and Bex. We all needed attention in different ways and we would often be told to listen and not to interrupt. Especially me. Bex and I talked about that recently

'I decided to ignore that piece of advice,' she said. 'Otherwise, I would never have got a word in edgeways.'

One time, Dad, sensing an audience, started to tell a story. It began to go on far too long and we were becoming restless.

Just as he was about to deliver the punchline, Mum quipped, 'Thank God that's over with.'

She got a huge laugh, which made Dad furious. Not only did he look like thunder, but Mum had stolen his thunder.

My little sister Bex and I were always close - I even remember Mum being pregnant with her and me helping Mum out of the chair when I was barely five. Bex and I have always got on and I make her laugh. I was more protective of her than of my next youngest sister Lu, who was always so capable - but she too is always game for a laugh.

At posh dinner parties, I would imitate an important guest without them seeing and Lu would fall about giggling and have to leave the room. Years later, when she was a qualified doctor, she suggested coming along with me to see my psychiatrist. As we entered the room, I said to the psychiatrist, an Indian gentleman:

'Hello, Doctor, do you mind if I bring my sister Lu along?'

'Certainly,' he replied, and then, looking at Lu, 'How long is it since he's been gone?'

'Been gone?' I muttered.

Lu and I keeled over with laughter. We both knew he meant to ask how long I had been unwell. The Doctor saw the funny side and added, in a strong accent, 'No, this is very healthy. Brother and sister laughing. Very healthy indeed.'

My Mum's parents lived on a farm. Her Mum was quite posh and had even been a debutante. My Uncle told me that before my Grandpa had won her over, she had been pursued across Europe by barons and counts. My grandparents had moved from London to live life in the country. For me and my older brother Tim especially, this was a place for adventure.Sometimes in the evenings, my Grandpa would take us out in the truck, tearing around the fields, looking for rabbits.

Bex and Lu would be upfront with him, calling out, 'There's one!'

And he'd shout out, in panic, 'Where? Damn and blast!'

Meanwhile, Tim and I would be ready at the back to shoot the stunned rabbits. Later, I remember skinning the rabbits with my Granny ready for the pot. That was holiday time.

When we first went to prep school, Tim and I had a routine. We had an intercom connecting our rooms. I would wake first and buzz him, 'Tim are you up?'

There'd be a muffled reply and he would make various noises to reassure me. 'Joe. Yeah, morning.'

And he'd lean over his bed and bang on the floor, imitating the sound of him padding about.Finally, we'd both make it downstairs and would take it in turns to cook breakfast. Tim would mostly do a fry up. I would make egg orange (orange juice with a whisked raw egg) and tea. We would then trek across West London to school together, sometimes in the dark, aged seven and eight.

Physically, we were like twins. The same height and weight for about ten years. That, combined with our competitive natures, encouraged us to push each other in sport, often overseen by Dad's keen eye. We became stronger and excelled. We played all sports and one year, Dad got us some boxing gloves, which we used on each other and our friends. We sometimes even had boxing birthday parties. Later in life, I joined a boxing club and with my newfound fitness, even ran a marathon.

Tim and I also had part-time jobs as paper boys and altar boys. The private quarters of the church felt mysterious and holy. We arrived early and put on our cassocks, awaiting instruction from the priest.

Once mass had begun, there were various duties to perform, including shutting the altar gate and guarding the entrance to the main holy altar area. This separated the priest and servers from the main congregation. It was my turn for that duty and I was quite nervous. The signal came from the priest and I went to try and lock the gate. But I couldn't fathom the latch so had to leave it closed, but not locked. I walked back to my seat feeling very uncomfortable. Later, one by one, the people queued to receive communion. The first person knelt before the gate and promptly fell straight through the doors onto the floor in front of the priest. I looked at Tim who was laughing hysterically. I was banned from serving for two weeks.

There was also an extra Mass on a Sunday, which was the 11.30. I was kneeling next to Tim at the altar. We were holding long candles while the priest gave the sermon.

'Joe,' Tim quietly said. 'We have to put out our hand on the altar for extra holiness.'

I duly complied, not knowing that putting your hand on the altar is a very serious offence. Only then did I notice Tim's hand had disappeared and that the priest was looking at me furiously.

'Tim, stop!' I shouted in a loud angry whisper. But he was laughing so much at his new naughtiness, he couldn't. I was banned again for another few weeks.

Our Dad on the other hand was mostly far better behaved. When singing, he would hold onto notes longer than anyone, In his rich actor's voice. He would often read the lesson at the pulpit, but when he wasn't reading, he would situate himself neither at the back with the old holy men, nor in the pews with the main congregation, but in the middle of the aisle towards the back, in a place of almost equal importance and prominence as the priest. Dad probably had his own feelings of grandeur.

As years went by, Mum became worried and exasperated by my sudden holiness, Dad was delighted while Tim, on the other hand, stopped going to church soon after leaving school. Looking back at my long history of mental health difficulties, I normally became more holy in the beginning or the middle of a nervous breakdown.

Despite my religious fervour, I never really understood the importance of reverence at church, nor the seriousness. I used to tease my sister, Lu, then about nine, about her first confession.

'Be careful,' I would say. 'The priest might poke you through the grill with a stick!'

She wouldn't find that funny at all.

I would also tease Bex, the youngest, and pretend to pray for her while we were next to each other in church.

'Dear Lord,' I would stage-whisper. 'Please forgive Becky for her terrible behaviour at breakfast this morning. I know she is a pain, but she doesn't realise it.'

My poor seven-year-old sister would feel mortified by this ticking off by her older brother, even more terrible for him bringing God into it.

The years passed. Tim grew up and began to take life a bit more seriously. I, meanwhile, struggled to behave and was regularly and severely punished. At my first big Catholic school, one female teacher smashed a recorder to pieces - over my head. I was seven. The head nun of my first school hit me across the face in a singularly humiliating way, in front of a class. I was only five and I realise now that I probably had undiagnosed ADHD.

Catholicism and naughtiness don't go together. I have found solace in my faith, although I don't attend Mass anymore. Guilt has a large part to play in my illness and most of that comes from the overbearing schooling and teachings of Catholic schools. In the end, I lost my mind and began to think I was Jesus and that continued off and on for nearly twenty-five years.

My last memory of Tim in our local Catholic church was about forty-five years ago. We were at the back and completely taken by surprise when a priest entered from a side door.

'Quick, Tim,' I said. 'A priest, look holy!'

We fell to our knees, did the sign of the cross and made a show of looking like we were deep in prayer.

I saw the Catholic mother of an old school friend recently and she came up to me and said, 'Oh, you and Timmy were such a couple of little Devils!'

Chapter 2
The beginning of illness
and the importance of friends

During my late teens, I gradually became unhinged. I had begun to struggle with relationships and the transition from boy to man. What I needed were the skills and tools to leave home, but I wasn't ready, or able. I was eighteen by now, working as a dispatch clerk for a publishing company during the week and a ten-hour day on a Saturday at a Marks and Spencer's warehouse. But even though I didn't know it, I was struggling mentally. My friends had gone to university, but I hadn't got the right A levels to get there, and the combination of these things was, I think, getting me down. Often, I found myself crying whilst on my motorbike on the way home from work. I was clashing with Mum, who had an uncanny ability to always be in the right.

I had lost Tim, who had gone to Bristol Uni a year earlier and was studying mechanical engineering. After a year or so, he saw me after the antidepressants had caused me to put on weight and the oil in them had caused an allergic reaction in my skin, which was a big change. We had been kids together, sporty, and always in good shape, so it was this physical change that was the biggest shock to him.

'What happened to Joe?' he asked.

But at that stage, I couldn't answer him because I was barely able to speak.

My Mum and Dad must have explained the situation to him and reassured him that I would get better because as far as I know, we all slept well that night. In the morning, I walked into Tim's room. He was barely awake. I picked up a fishing net and placed it on his head, as though I was knighting him. With a great deal of effort, I mustered up some words.

'You are probably the best mechanical engineer the world has ever seen,' I said.

I then left the net on his head and calmly exited his room, leaving him with a startled and sleepy expression.

Sometime later, Tim said to me, ``What was so funny about that, was that I was probably the worst mechanical engineer in the world.'

Recovering from mental illness needs a lot of love and understanding but many other things too including loyalty, kindness, and compassion, not just from family, but from friends as well. I have four great friends that I have known for about fifty years. A bond that stands the test of time. With all my friends, comes a degree of bravery and an ability to laugh at themselves. Their names are Matt, John, Jay, and Ben, although, later, in my religious delusion, I would come to know them as Matthew, Mark, Luke, and John.

I can't remember moving into our house in Barnes but do remember meeting my new best friend Matt. I was four. Mum and I were on our way round the block to meet her friend, Ruth.

I looked up at the clouds and asked, 'Do the clouds go faster than a plane?'

'Oh, I expect so.'
'How fast is that?'
'Oh, hundreds of miles an hour.'
'But they don't seem to go that fast when I look at them.'
Mum changed the subject and told me we were also meeting Ruth's children, Matt and Claire, who she said were twins.

What a strange word, I thought and hoped they were mostly human.

I remember getting on very well with Matt from the off. From an early age, we would encourage and complement each other and would find each other funny. Once, we nicked our arms with a penknife and pushed our arms together to cement our friendship: blood brothers.

Matt also loved to have fun and was imaginative. He converted his garage into a place of adventure, and we formed our secret gang with codewords. In the school holidays, Jay would be around too, and we all became great mates.

We remained friends right up until young adulthood and beyond. Matt showed real insight and wisdom when I first got ill. In that respect, he was wise beyond his years. He would often visit me and listen to my deluded thoughts rather than say:

'That's a load of old crap,' or 'Joe, I don't think so.'

He would almost get drawn in by my madness and find logic to it, albeit tenuous. This patience and understanding were very helpful to me and in time I would recover enough and work my way around to normal ideas and thought patterns.

One visit was a disaster. He arrived and I almost immediately challenged him to a game of table tennis. He refused and so I arranged the furniture like a Roman Colosseum and challenged Matt to a fight.

'I don't want to fight you, you're my friend,' he shouted at me.

I was determined but Matt must have walked away or managed to diffuse the situation. Later, I can remember feeling ashamed. He was my best friend. What the hell had I been thinking?

At that moment, I think I knew I needed help and I was in the right place for it.

There was also a sensitive side to Matt and we liked to talk, even before I became ill and sometimes at great length too. Our Mums would laugh at these two teenagers putting the world to rights.

A few years later, he experienced problems at sixth-form college – fallings out with tutors and difficulties deciding whether to stay on or not. I helped him during this time and we seemed closer than ever. He was surprised at my understanding of what he was going through. However, about a year later, it was Matt helping me. He knew I was having a nervous breakdown before anyone else outside my family. He was sensitive and mature in the face of my increasing paranoia, which sometimes manifested itself in thinking that he, or anyone who told me I looked well, wanted to sleep with me. I feel very embarrassed remembering this now, as there was nothing but friendship between Matt and myself, but that's how it was. Many people think that paranoia is thinking that everyone is against you when sometimes it's thinking everyone loves you!

Matt was only eighteen, but he still handled it well. When I became increasingly angry and defensive, when I wouldn't listen to anyone who tried to tell me I was losing my mind, he said it was so sad to see me get so ill in my prime. After the breakdown, I was more vulnerable and this was difficult for him. I was now looking up to him, rather than the other way around, like a reversal of roles. But he stepped up and was there all the way through.

Half a lifetime later and we're still close. He lives in Brighton with his wife and has two grown-up children. He said recently that my illness had inspired him to take up psychotherapy as a career. He's perfect for the job as he's wise, interested and has a lot of experience. He does have a sad side too and sometimes an inability to return phone calls.

'Sorry I haven't been in touch, Joe,' he said to me recently. 'I've been in a dark space.'

I said, 'You haven't been up in that attic again, have you?'

The friend that I have known the longest is Ben. I've known him all my life and we were even in prams together. His Mum and my Mum are also great friends. Ben's Mum, my Mum's best friend, Sylvia Syms, gained an MBE for her services to acting and charity. As a child, I would sometimes mistake her for my Mum, because of her blonde hair.

Ben was always very daring, and he was the first child in the neighbourhood to ride his Raleigh Chopper, the iconic 1970s bike modelled in the style of a Harley Davidson. He would give me 'backies'- I would hang on desperately to the back of the seat as he zoomed round corners like a daredevil.

Later they moved to Cobham and we lost touch for a while. He soon progressed to real motorbikes and, like me, he rebelled and began to live an unorthodox and risky lifestyle. He joined a bike gang and got into fights. A while ago, we went to Cobham to look at some of his old haunts and he showed me where some of his biker mates would hang out. It was as much fun being on the back of his motorbike as it had been on the back of the pushbike. He wasn't a kid anymore, but he was still just as daring. Once, we were doing seventy miles an hour and he suddenly ducked down low over the crossbar, and I nearly got blown off by the power of the wind. It hit me like a punch.

'What the fuck are you doing?' I shouted at him.

He knew exactly what he was doing and was now giggling at his devilishness. His laugh was infectious.

Ben is widely travelled and can speak five languages. I remember about thirty-five years ago, Ben visited me in hospital. I was recovering from an overdose and was attached to a drip. This shows how our paths would so often cross and sometimes in such sad situations. I was touched by his visit. Months went by and I was in hospital again. This time it was a psychiatric hospital. Yet again, his loyalty prevailed. He was on the run from the police and managed to come and see me, on his motorbike, despite his hectic schedule!

'Here's a tenner,' he said, thrusting a note at me. ' Get yourself some baccy and some coffee, I know what it's like in here.'

I was surprised and delighted to see him. We spoke about boxing in the old days and his visit rekindled my interest. A year later, I joined a boxing club.

He was always popular with women and my girlfriend's Mum asked me recently whether he had a wife. I thought she said bike.

'I think he's got one in Bangkok,' I said, 'and I know he keeps one in the shed.'

Jay is a treasured conundrum. On the one hand, he can be elusive and private, but on the other, your best mate. He moved into the neighbourhood when he was six and I was seven. We immediately began competing. Indoors, it could be table football or table tennis. Or we would be outside kicking a ball around. It laid down the foundations for a lifelong friendship. At the time, all the activity toughened us up and kept us fit. As we got older, sports remained close to our hearts and we began to enjoy cricket and golf and even fishing.

Jay began to shine at cricket, and I remember standing at the bar of his cricket club when a stranger approached me.

'Do you know where I can find the captain of the first team?' he said.

'Yes,' I said, 'He's over there on the floor.'

Jay was indeed on the floor, waving his feet in the air, tipsy and without a care in the world.

We had many holidays together and many camping trips too, which we would combine with fishing and golf. One campsite we stayed at had a sign on the gate: *Couples and families only*. Which made us both laugh. I rang up Matt in our merriment.

He laughed too and said, 'You two are like an old couple anyway.'

Sometimes Jay would get out of his tent at dawn and find me warming myself up in the heat of the car! It was a huge shock to Jay when I became ill. It was Jay who walked past me in Ladbroke Grove that day I had my first dramatic breakdown. In my Jesus delusion, I called out to him:

'Hey, is your name Mark or Luke?'

He walked past. We've never really spoken about it, but I know he will have been so shocked. We were still teenagers after all. Over time, he did grow to understand and has remained a great friend to this day. He copes with humour, sometimes imitating the way I walk after an injection or a brain scan, which will make me fall about laughing. We still make each other laugh and we still go fishing and play golf together.

I met John at my first big Catholic school, St. Benedict's, aged seven. We were in the same class together and got on well. However, we both tended to misbehave. At the age of seven and during the first term at school, a female class teacher said,

'Oh Joby, you're such a cheeky monkey.' Joby was my childhood name, from my middle name, Job.

I replied, 'You're a big, fat, hairy gorilla.'

I was consequently marched up to the headmaster's office. John thought this was brilliant and virtually ran home to tell his folks.

Soon, John and a few of us were asked to keep a diary. I think it was to keep us focused and we struggled on and up to the middle school, where we found ourselves in the bottom stream. John was bright though and I think his dyslexia played a part in his academic mediocrity. I could never understand my academic weakness, although later found out that I had a form of ADHD and that's perhaps why I was interrupting lessons and showing off.

John always felt like an older brother who was looking after me. Sometimes he would jump back on a train we'd just got off to rescue a bag that I may have forgotten. Or he'd even sacrifice himself at school and take a punishment for me. He was fiercely loyal and over a big span of years we stayed close and still are to this day – I meet him most weeks for lunch and whilst he is a little more serious these days, he is still a lot of fun. He'd already gone to Uni by the time I became very ill but when he describes that time, he says:

'Joe, your brain chemistry was all over the place.'

Which it was.

Chapter 3
My first breakdown

1980. I was eighteen. I was working as a dispatch clerk for a financial publisher. One afternoon, I left my desk and walked out of the office, not before flicking the tie of the Managing Director by way of goodbye.

I was now outside. I had broken free from the constraints of work, good behaviour and sanity. I stripped off to the waist and began to walk in the middle of the road, holding up traffic. I found myself beside some railings, next to Latimer Road train station, in West London. I gripped onto the railings and began shouting at the cars.... cheering the clean colourful ones and jeering at the dirty ones. They, I thought, represented the devil.

Half an hour passed, although I wasn't aware of time. A fair size contingent of police arrived in a van and began engaging with me directly. They addressed me by my name. Some of them were around corners on walkie-talkies, my sister Lu later told me.

I was still holding onto the railings, still stripped to the waist. There was a gash on my back from the night before, from where I had been drunk and fallen and I can remember thinking that the railings were at the same height as my injury and that this was a good reason to hold onto them.

Lu was there with my Dad, and they pleaded with me to come home.

'Joe,' she said. She was crying. 'It's OK, Joe. You can come with us now.'

I can't remember if my Dad said anything. If he did, it would have been roughly the same thing. Both would have been desperate for me to come with them. I refused.

'Not until the whole of Ladbroke Grove follows me home on the white lines, 'I called out to them.'The ones in the middle of the road.'

During all this commotion, I had been piecing facts together, in a disorderly fashion. It was like I was trying to make sense of a jumbled-up jigsaw puzzle. Eventually, I was persuaded into the van.

The British police were the best in the world and my family and friends were the best anyone could have too. I had three friends. Mathew, Ben and John, so my other friend, according to the Bible, must be Mark or Luke. At that very moment, Jay passed me, as he worked nearby, and I asked him if his name was Mark, or Luke. He smiled, embarrassed, and continued. That's when I knew I was Jesus.

I eventually agreed to go down to the local police station, while they decided what to do with me...I was taken to a psychiatric hospital in Epsom called Longrove. During the first month, I became worse, going from aggression, grandiose ideas and psychosis to feelings of anxiety and loss of freedom. I was getting signs from the television and began smoking heavily. I was also getting confusing signs, from the direction someone's foot was pointing, or from a knowing smile at the end of a room. It could all have a hidden meaning that I would interpret, usually wrongly.

I began following a black cat, which represented both my girlfriend at the time, Zoe, and God. My confusion was at its worst. In my mind, everyone I met was the best in the world at something: incoherent old men were the funniest in the world; odd, elderly women were in the Mafia and young disturbed people were the cleverest brains or world leaders. I was having a type of religious breakdown, suffering psychotic delusions. I felt that I had to go through the humiliation and sacrifice myself to God.

One night, I was in the kitchen and began purifying myself with water. I left the room and collided with a man who was carrying a teapot. This seemed to be the right moment for my humiliation. I stripped naked and stood in front of the television with my arms outstretched in a pose of a crucifix. The staff carried me to a room and I noticed that they had prepared an injection for me, which was going to be put into a vein in my arm. I thought it was meant to kill me and I was terrified. I was held down and I can't remember anything anyone said but I remember that one nurse smiled at me, aware of the fear in my eyes, which eased my pain momentarily. I felt like he cared about me and that softened the situation.

The injection was an antipsychotic tranquilliser. Shortly afterwards, I was allowed outside the room and I noticed the cat was opposite, sitting on a window ledge. The cat at that moment represented God and I was reassured. God was there with me, protecting me. The cat then jumped out of the window. It felt like God was deserting me and I was being left to face the Devil alone. I fainted in terror.

I was in that hospital for three or four months. When I came out, I was on strong medication – a lot of pills, plus I had to go to a hospital in Richmond for regular injections and attend a day centre each day. I did this off and on for many years and met many friends there.

A year or two later, I was in hospital again though this time, it was less severe. Once again, I found myself dealing with God. Although I was naked again, I had formed an orderly queue in the hospital church and was calmly preparing to receive communion. Looking back, I find this funny and I think even then, in my late teens, I probably thought it was hilarious. I always liked to make my friends laugh and enjoyed making a spectacle, but I can see now that I had gone to extremes and had lost all sense of decorum and appropriate behaviour.

A nurse must have shouted at me and wrestled me to the floor. I remember that the priest stopped the mass while this commotion was going on.

The nurse agreed to leave me if I dressed. Which I did. Oh well, I thought. What shall I do now?

In my mind, what had happened was no big deal. Sometimes I think that being treated like a 'nutter' made me behave like one. I also wonder whether I was simply bored and in need of some, any, entertainment. I wanted drama.

I was in a less secure ward. In my search for something to do, I decided I would venture out. I did this quite frequently. I might wander off into Epsom via roads and fields, meeting all manner of people along the way.

'You can't go there, mate,' someone might say to me if I was walking through their garden or, 'Excuse me sir, can I help you?' if I'd wandered into a shop.

I wasn't aware of where I was going or what I was doing. Most of the time, I kept to myself and would be at nature's beckoning – falling leaves might tell me where to go, the wind, the trees. Confused, I would continue with no other aim but to press on. A signpost might say something like, London A3 10 Miles.

That's a trick, I would think. I'll go this way instead.

Epsom 4 Miles!

That's another trick I thought.

Looking back, I'm surprised that I wasn't going around in circles. As it was, I would sometimes be picked up by the police who would take me back to the hospital, or I would find my way back on my own on foot or by bus.

The most romantic of these adventures came one morning when a young woman and I were passing the time of day and were in a similar frame of mind. I asked her if she'd like to go out.

'Where would we go?'

'Let's get on a bus and see what happens.'

'What might happen if we get on a bus?'

Before pondering too long, we were on our way. I remember at one point being trapped in a field of horses and being separated by them, but we managed to manoeuvre our way out of the field safely. We trekked across the countryside and ended up by Epsom Downs and had a peaceful drink in a pub. After a while, we also both noticed it was getting late and decided to make our way back.

We stopped by a meadow in full bloom. The sun was setting, and I asked her if she was happy.

'Yes,' she said. 'Are you?' 'Yes.'

We leaned together to kiss. It felt magical and romantic and soon, arm in arm, we returned safely to the hospital. That is one of my happier memories.

After my first six-month section was nearly over and when I was allowed home. Dad had come to pick me up. I said my goodbyes and said to him 'This is the best day of my life.'Dad replied,

'That will be when you are completely better.'

Chapter 4
Edward de Souza

During the Cold War in the late 1950s, Mum and Dad, as part of a drama company, had gone on a cultural exchange with a Russian ballet school. It was exciting, and they didn't know what to expect. At that moment in time, it was like going to the moon. As soon as they were off the plane, the first people Dad met were twins and he thought.

'Crikey, these Russians all look the same.'

My first memories of Dad were of a big, hugging, loveable man. I soon realised he wasn't in a normal job and he wasn't your average man. He had a successful career as an actor and had a talent for watercolour paintings, DIY, and sport.

He would be great at playing games with the children, especially 'sleeping lions.' He would pretend to be asleep and we would all sneak up on him and suddenly he would wake up and bellow and roar and chase us around the house.

Not only was he good at sport, but he would be keen on helping me and my brother Tim to become good all-rounders. He gave us a set of weights when we were aged twelve or thirteen and we also used to box under his supervision. We would compete at chins to the bar and he would insist that we 'breathe' each time we reached the bar. I also noticed that he would do this same breathing technique in the kitchen when he picked up the kettle.

He was a good driver, if not a little eccentric. Everything seemed to be in slow motion, and he would give slow thank you, hand signals to people down side roads who seemed to have nothing to do with us. He once told me he was the slowest walker at Rada.

Sunday lunch was a palaver. Mum would be rushing around trying to get everything ready, while Dad took his time sharpening the knife and carving. He was never in a rush and quite often Mum would be hurrying him up and he would say,

'I am just finishing my coffee!'

Once, there was a DIY job to do and he was halfway up a ladder when Mum passed him something and Dad, being in an awkward position, replied,

'Darling, I am at the Zenith of my discomfort!'

Dad was full of odd behaviours. Once, my Mum sent him and I on an errand to sort out *Joe's sock situation*. I brought along a great friend and it was a nice outing. What was unusual was the fact that Dad was now in charge of my socks. We arrived in Hammersmith and duly found the sock counter. Within a split second of arriving there, he was on his hands and knees and announced as if he was giving a speech:

'Right, what we have here is socks and what we've got to do...' he paused and took a deep breath, 'is to differentiate between the socks we have here and the socks we have at home!'

My friend moved off to the food counter.

If Mum's friend Sylvia dropped by, Dad would rush into the living room and pretend to be asleep. Mum would usher her friend into the kitchen, and we could hear him 'snoring' next door. Another time, we were in the garden one summer's day and suddenly he announced:

'Bees aren't designed to fly.'

And Sylvia piped up, 'There's one,' and pointed to a bee flying by. Later, he appeared to be furious and said,

'Didn't she have any idea what I meant by that?'

I knew what he'd meant – that bees' bodies seem too fat for their tiny wings – but I was confused as to why he was so angry. Sometimes, he was baffling.

He could create tension, but he was also good at diffusing a stressful situation. One summer, for example, I had arranged a boating holiday up the Thames with my girlfriend and my two best mates. Dad had agreed to take us to the pickup point. We appeared to be a little lost, but far from being worried himself, he pointed out an odd-looking character and said:

'He won't know the way.'

Which got us all giggling.

He too had gone on a boating holiday many years before, but on his own. Having arrived at a small country village and having had a few beers, he was surprised to find it deserted. Somehow, on his travels, he had lost a day and had arrived not on Saturday but a 'sleepy Sunday.'

Dad was still energetic and active at eighty and was still good at golf. Although after years of playing once a week, we began using a buggy, which he would drive like he would a car, or like someone being watched in a driving test, threading the wheel through his hands and moving very slowly. When we had got just far enough ahead of the group behind, he often stopped and rolled a leisurely cigarette.

We played in all weathers and enjoyed stopping off at the mobile van for a chance to have a cuppa and catch up with other golfers. If he didn't like the look of someone's trousers, he might announce,

'I don't like your tailor.' Or 'Your putter is illegal!'

They would look at worst offended and at best bemused. My father's good looks and stature, as well as his actor's projection, meant that he would usually get away with it.

If a pair behind us politely asked to play through, he would often tell them he would be delighted, as he could learn a lot from watching their behinds.

Once, he walked purposefully beyond the mobile café and in front of everyone, laid down on the floor. Even to my surprise, several golfers began to look concerned and one man asked if he was OK.

'I think he's lining up a putt,' I said – a golfer's joke. He was trying to cure his hiccups.

Other times, he might charge across the fairway to talk to a complete stranger, if the mood took him and often would behave in a far from regular way, breaking normal golf etiquette. After a while, other golfers might ask if he was an actor - possibly because he was behaving so strangely and funnily, or possibly because they had recognized him.

I grew up watching him on TV and going to watch him in plays and in more recent years, he became well-known on the radio in *The Man in Black* and I was always proud of him. He came to watch my brother Tim and I play rugby and coined a new phrase.

'Eight men, eight men,' he would call out.

Nobody was quite sure what it meant.

But before he reached the action you could see him walking towards the game ever so slowly with a roll up paper stuck to his bottom lip. Even that was a bit of a performance. You would think he would have been banned for all these eccentricities but in fact, he was the only Dad invited to the rugby dinner and we all loved him.

Chapter 5
Longrove and Horton hospitals

After I was delivered to the Psychiatric hospital Long Grove, for the first time, I was greeted by a funny-looking man, wearing a funny-looking tie. It seemed to me that this whole place, the people in it and me, were all part of a big façade. Everybody knows that I'm Jesus, I thought, so why have I been placed here by the police? I connected everything and everybody inaccurately and my visitors would be frustrated by my strange connections.

'See that man over there,' I would say. 'He's the cleverest and wisest man in England.'

'No, he's not,' my sister Becky would reply. 'He just hasn't shaved for a month,'

I would walk around looking for people to heal, which wasn't difficult, as they all liked the attention. I would lay my hand on an old lady's swollen ankle, for example, and adopt a holy, yet expressionless face. I'm not sure if I said anything to these people or if I asked permission. I can't remember how they reacted, but I suppose they must have let me get on with it.

The initial lock up, when I was sectioned at eighteen, was in the far wing of Longrove. It was called Southview Villa. It was locked and the staff were highly trained. I was there for three months, but after the first weeks, I was allowed into the hospital grounds. This meant I would often go to the social centre.

There was a general medley of characters from all around, where we would congregate and it was there that I found one or two very old, foreign patients, from Eastern Europe, who had been in the hospital since the war. They still couldn't speak English; would wear their war medals and they stuck together in a small group. Other small groups would hang out together in hierarchical order – they would play competitive card games, drafts, chess, table tennis, and at tea break, a door would open and there would be about fifty cups of tea lined up and ready. Some of the patients would run to get their tea first.

I remember seeing them and not thinking that I was any different to them in any way. Perhaps they were normal to me, by then.

There was a man called John, who thought he was the King of England and when he wasn't rolling around on the floor, would break a ciggy into three and would sell each bit individually. He would also sell a teaspoon of his coffee from a jar that he would carry around with him. We once both went looking for an apple in a field nearby and ended up near a gypsy caravan until a man came to the door of the van.

'Oi,' he shouted at us. 'What the bloody hell do you think you're doing?'

'We've come for an apple,' we explained.

He wasn't impressed. We got very short shrift and retreated to the hospital – without the apple.

The grounds surrounding Longrove were beautiful; great trees, and shrubbery and easy access into the surrounding countryside, which was home to wild deer, and I would often roam freely. I met an Italian woman from the ward, and we would sometimes go for long walks and end up making love in the great outdoors. Those are happy memories for me. But I would also sometimes escape on my own and find myself miles away. I couldn't access money in hospital, nor at my local branch, but I would get myself to the Epsom branch and cash cheques. I once managed to get to Liverpool by train in my slippers. I suppose this must have attracted attention and I got mugged – not violently, as I was quite happy to hand over my money. That time, despite being robbed on the way, I stayed the night in a youth hostel.

The thing is, at times like this, I never really had a plan. I never knew where I was going or why, I just went. I was on strong medication, but I hadn't accepted that it could help me in any way. And when I went on my adventures, I stopped taking the medication, which can't have been ideal, although it was mostly only one day and one night. I often returned on my own – sometimes hitching lifts. They would ask me where I was going and sometimes, I would say I didn't know so they would contact the police. Once the police found me and I told them I was at Longrove. They contacted Longrove and Longrove sent a car – even though I was miles away.

On my return, it was back to the old routine. The hospital was connected by endless corridors and as many different wards. There were day shifts and night shifts and the catering staff and a social centre for the staff (which we could never get into). There was also a patient's bank and you could withdraw small amounts of money for things like tobacco. There would be a small gathering in the evening with the night nurses and we would play bingo for prizes like shampoo. Thinking about that now, I realise I must have been institutionalised – I liked many of the nurses and the other patients and I enjoyed playing bingo and would be delighted to win a bubble bath.

In the mornings, there would sometimes be communal bath time, which didn't seem weird to me at that time. Turns were taken and there were four baths alongside each other. A jug of water would sometimes be encouragingly dispensed onto a hapless patient's head and as soon as that was over, we would be shaved – we weren't allowed razors, of course. I was only a teenager and on one visit, I asked Dad in which order the three s's should be taken and we both seemed to agree; shit, shower and then shave. I took this advice very seriously.

Many patients, including me, didn't like taking medication. Partly because they didn't think there was anything wrong with them and partly because of their grandiose idea

'I am Napoleon. Or Jesus. Why on earth should I take these silly pills?'

I was transferred to another local hospital, Horton, along with some other young men. By this time, I was twenty-three. They used a van to move us and presumably, we all had a ward allocated to us.

I remember when we had got out of the van, being singled out, as I was acting up and a few of the male nurses had surrounded me. I ran as fast as I could, but soon enough they caught up with me and I went peacefully. This time, I went to a more acute ward and in time, I intuitively began to sense that I should behave as well as I could, so that I could get to a less severe ward and so closer to freedom.

So, during a ward round, I became serious about putting myself forward in the most presentable manner possible. There was a gathering of nurses, doctors and social workers present and I remember thinking it was going well. Finally, as I was about to leave, the main ward psychiatrist asked if I had anything to add.

'Yes,' I said. 'There is one thing. Every time I take a step forward, I think I'm being carried by hundreds of ants.'

I remember saying that very vividly and I can't believe I thought that was a reasonable thing to say. I was sane enough to realize that I had to try and behave 'normally' but not sane enough to know how to do that. I genuinely thought that I was acting 'normal'.

I met some colourful people and learned some lessons and in time began to recover. After a period spent in halfway houses, I managed to get my own place with a housing trust, although I was still in touch with some of my friends from the hospital.

One dawn morning, around five a.m. I got a knock on the door. It was Rich. A man that I had been locked up with. I opened the door and there he was, a tall figure in front of me. He had a pair of dungarees on, which barely covered his knees, a funny pair of plimsolls and a child's baseball cap, turned sideways on top of his long Rastafarian, flowing locks. He was also holding a miniature tennis racket.

'Hi Joe,' he said. 'Fancy a game of tennis?'

'I haven't got a spare tennis racket,' I said. 'But come in and have a cuppa.'

Later, I introduced Rich to Mum, who immediately asked:

'Hello, Rich, do you live nearby?'

'I'm just out of hospital.'
'Oh dear, where's your mother?'
'She's in Holloway.'
'Oh lovely, is that a nice area?'

Chapter 6
The Escape

I had many escapes, as I've said but this one was the biggest. It was Nineteen Eighty and I was eighteen years old. I was in Longrove psychiatric hospital in Epsom and had been locked up in the secure unit for approximately one month. I had been transferred from a less acute ward and was moved to a more severe unit for my safety and the safety of others.

Patients were kept inside at night. It was a scary and daunting place. Not only because of the people inside but also because there was no privacy. The bed space was partitioned by meagre plywood. The only private area was a secure room, which in effect was a lock up room within a lock up ward. I noticed at the end of this room was a Perspex window.

'Was it secure?' I asked myself.

The nurses were segregated and had their own room. Once, with pure frustration at needing to talk to them, I yanked the entire door handle off its hinges.

In the morning we were woken up, sometimes boisterously by the staff. One man who often didn't want to get out of bed, was literally tipped out of his bed onto the floor. We were led into the bathrooms for washing and shaving before breakfast. It was a million miles away from studying at college and with my first proper job a few months earlier.

Time passed and I became used to the routine. My Mum was concerned that I was becoming institutionalised. I understood what she meant, although I couldn't pretend to be better than I was.

'Darling, do try to get better. You've been here ages. Try to get back to Southview villa.'

That was the less severe ward that I had originally come from. Dad joined in;

'Yes, Joe, when you get back there, you could play ping pong and I could bring you a few golf clubs ...' (There was a field nearby)

I thought that was a good idea and a feeling of warmth and hope filled my stomach. It was lovely to see them and with renewed vigour, I continued.

The strangest thing about being ill, is that you don't think you are. The doctors, nurses and your family and friends all seem to be playing along.

Sometimes visitors were turned away by the staff, as I was too ill to be seen. On the other hand, visits could be entertaining. Once, I insisted that everyone had to spin around three hundred and sixty degrees before they sat down, if they hadn't already turned left, whilst entering the room.

Visits would often be a mecca for other patients vying for attention. Visitors would be asked for lifts from patients even though they may be in their pyjamas. There were also endless cups of tea and coffee made and drunk at visiting times. On one visit, I asked an ill friend of mine to pretend to be a psychiatrist and introduce himself to my Mum. We knew she was coming, and I described her to him. Sure enough, she entered the room and Rod took his chance. At least he didn't believe he was a doctor and agreed to play along.

'Hello, Madam, very pleased to meet you. My name is Doctor Stevenson, how can I help you?'

Rod was limping and he was looking particularly scruffy, with unkempt hair and odd oversized glasses, but Mum couldn't be completely sure.

'Yes, I've come to see Joe'

He left Mum and clumsily crashed into a chair on his way out, before returning with me and then successfully exiting. This left Mum with a surprised expression and she said, 'What a very peculiar psychiatrist.'

Mum and I chatted for a while and various patients came to talk to us, including one or two from the women's ward. It was lovely to see her and I was sad to see her go.

We were connected to the female dormitory through a corridor, interlinking both wards and by a large wooden door. When it was open, there would be an intermittent flow, both into the women's dorm and vice versa. I met a woman called Lucy. She had shoulder-length brown hair and was Italian. Despite the morose buildings of the hospital, the local landscape was beautiful, although it was sometime before we were allowed out together.

After seeing Mum and with the combination of my frustrating lack of freedom, I decided that I would try and escape. Patients were milling around and I went to take another look at the window in the lock-up room. I noticed that there were two pieces of Perspex with a gap in-between. At the top of each piece was a large gap and both pieces of the Perspex could be slid upwards and so leaving space at the bottom to climb through. I sensed my chance and I knew that I could just do it. I managed to find a chair. I stepped up onto it, which left me high enough to begin to climb through. I raised the first piece and with most of my weight on the chair, I climbed through the gap. I lifted the second piece and nimbly squeezed through and was out. I climbed down onto the roof, down a drainpipe and like a cat burglar, I stole into the night.

I was still battling a war against the Devil and in my mind, Jesus was winning. I was totally confused. Any road signs that I saw were undoubtedly contaminated by the Devil, just to confuse me. So, if a sign pointed me in one direction, I would turn and walk in another. Not only that, I felt that God was helping me during my escape. He was guiding me in the direction that I should be going. That took the form of visual hallucinations, clouds in the sky forming shapes, a gust of wind, and even a branch of a tree pointing in a direction for me to follow. I would also take a good look at cars passing by and would find a message through the colour or the number plate. I would be climbing over fences, through fields, paths and by road. I was being torn one way by God and one way by the Devil and neither of them were doing any good. I should have been in the relative safety of the hospital.

Not only was I completely lost, but I was also quite mad.

Chapter 7

The rabbits and the gun

I was on my grandparents' farm and I was nineteen. I sat motionless. I was on a grass verge, inside a tunnel of trees. It was dusk and the rabbits were beginning to appear from their warrens to feed and frolic. The shotgun was positioned directly across my lap, aimed in the direction of the rabbits, as they appeared one by one.

'Go and get one for supper,' my grandpa had said.

Time stood still. I sat a few hundred metres from the farmhouse until it was nearly dark. My arm hadn't risen to shoot. Instead, I was enjoying the rare moment of peace and quiet, which was only interrupted by the chorus of the night singing from the birds.

As I sat in the grounds of my grandparents' farm, the gun held a strange comfort for me. That night I didn't want to shoot any rabbits, but I did think of shooting myself.

I turned the gun to my temple. While the gun was aimed directly at my head, I sat there as still as death. Minutes passed.

Eventually, I was called in by my grandpa.

'Joe, time to come in.' He leaned out of the window and shouted across the field.

I got up and made the short walk across the meadow to the house. Walking purposefully, the gun pointing down safely, just like he had taught me.

Chapter 8

The waiting room

I was in and out of hospital throughout my twenties. One time, I arrived at the hospital and went straight to reception. 'Busy?' I asked, and was told:

'There's a steady flow.'

Good, not long to wait, I thought.

When I got to the waiting room, seats were scarce. So, I placed myself in between a heavily drugged man and a strong-looking man who told me he was a builder. I asked him what he was waiting for.

'There's nothing wrong with me,' he said. 'I'm late for work.'

He was there for help, like me, but this is the kind of conversation that would happen in those waiting rooms.I continued to chat with him and he told me he was worried about one of the side effects of the pills.

'Oh dear, 'I said. 'What's that?'

'Death,' he said.

Although what he was most upset by was that he had been trapped in a system against his will and all he had done was open the gate for an old lady.

That's when the oddest man joined in. He had bulged eyes and his face was sunken and he had long lifeless hair drooping below his shoulders. He too found it extraordinary to find himself in this position and began to talk quite eloquently to the builder about their situation.

'Do you realise I've been in this predicament for thirty-three years?' he began.

'You poor sod. ' Replied the builder.

'There was a stage when I was completely medication free.'

'When was that?'

'It was a brief period before I was put on a six-month section.'

The builder went a little quiet.

Then, two new patients arrived and suddenly there was an impatience to be seen. One man moved towards the door and was told to get back in the queue.

'I was only looking at the notice board.' he said.

There was a jostling of positions and arguments about who was next. One man shouted out:

'I've been here since Tuesday.'

The injection room opened, and the nurse apologised and asked us for our patience. That's when one of the men who had just walked in got on his knees and began to pray.

Then the injection room door sprang open and the heavily drugged man, who hadn't spoken at all, and the builder, rushed to the door and the quiet man said in a loud and clear voice

'This simply won't do.'

And the builder replied, 'You're all fucking nuts and I need to get out of here.'

There was a scuffle at the entrance to the room and a picture on the wall was dislodged and smashed on the floor.

The disturbance was quelled, and I entered the injection room to find the nurse on the phone to security.

All I could hear was: 'Smashed. Yes. An imitation Van Gough.'

Crisis over, the nurse asked me some basic questions, including how long I had been at the hospital.

I replied, 'Thirty-four years. Amazing, isn't it?'

She seemed to ignore that and was concentrating on drawing up the injection. She then gave me the intramuscular injection into my backside.

I said, 'Ah, that's better.' Which was nonsense because it was a slow-release medication designed to function over weeks.

But as she was withdrawing the needle, I let out a small amount of wind. Thankfully, she didn't say anything. As I buttoned myself up and politely said my farewell, I noticed that there was no eye contact and her face had turned into a grimace.

Chapter 9

The highs, the lows
and the funny side of grandiosity

Before my son came along, my life was a series of big ups and downs, which always ended up with me being hospitalised.

I would fester in hospital, sometimes for months. A social worker once told me the natural cycle of a breakdown is around two months. Often, you have reached the point of crisis before you are admitted but deteriorate further while you are in hospital. I would challenge my section, but by that point, it showed I was nearly ready for release and so that route was futile, as I was now tentatively being let off the hook.

Even so, it was always a great relief to see the outside world and get my first taste of freedom. I was allowed off the leash, only to be pulled back in if I didn't stick to the rules. I was allowed out two hours a week at first, if accompanied by a nurse or a responsible visitor. Then, bit by bit, I was let out for the occasional hour on my own – a trip to the local shop or a walk around the park.

After a few weeks, as my progress continued, I wouldn't feel the need to escape, because I knew it would jeopardise my chances of release. This aspect of serious mental illness forms a kind of loop: you pretend to be better than you are to reach a less acute ward and eventually be released altogether. However, in all the years of hospitalisation, I never felt like they kept me in longer than I needed to inside.

In one hospital, when I was first allowed out, a peculiar male nurse accompanied me. I found it surprising that he agreed that I was Jesus and we prayed together. Even in my confused state, it occurred to me that he was a bit odd and maybe everyone from that hospital was a bit cuckoo, including the staff.

I can remember on one occasion I was allowed out on my own and around the corner from the hospital was Tolworth high street. After so long in hospital, it seemed like a magical mystery tour. Every new sight and sound, even the smells were exciting. All the shops looked fascinating and going into them, even more so. I had little money and what I did spend, I did very carefully, on rubbish. I had become rusty at spending on anything useful. Although I had my first pint of beer in ages and savoured it.

In the hospital, cash and tobacco were always in short supply. Apart from the occasional telephone call, what else could I spend a meagre few shillings on? Except for tobacco. When I had no money or cigarettes, I even took to rummaging around all the ashtrays in the main room, stocking up on dog ends. Once, when I did have some baccy, a fellow patient ran off with it. I never did find out where he had hidden it.

There were often one or two familiar faces I would know, whether in the lockups, or less severe wards. For example, Ned, and I were often in the same ward and we even got transferred together to a less acute ward.

Each time I got out, I needed to go through the process of becoming self-sufficient again. The whole business of paying bills and buying food was there to be learnt all over again. Even my driving was ropey, as I hadn't been permitted to, or been safe enough whilst sectioned. When I got ill, my car keys were confiscated and that was that.

However, there was an occasion when I had planned to drive up to Scotland in the middle of the night. I was so paranoid and thought that unmarked police cars were following me. I took several diversions to throw them off the scent but only ended up as far as Milton Keynes. I decided to turn back and ended up in a church in North London. In a moment of grandiosity, I decided to donate my car to the church. I parked my car perfectly, went inside and placed my car keys in the congregation box. I then left the church and went to the nearest hospital and phoned my parents.

'Joe!' my Mum answered, worried sick. 'Where are you?'

'North London,' I told her. 'I've given my car to the church.'

She eventually got a road name and the name of the hospital out of me and she and my father drove to the church. My keys were eventually found in the congregation box by a very surprised priest and returned to my exasperated parents.

Later that night, I was moved to a mental hospital in Epsom and stayed there for a few weeks or months, I can't remember exactly. I always felt safe at Epsom.

So, my friendships moved between my old 'well' friends and my new, not-so-well friends. My Dad would describe them as,' not complete.' I brought one friend home unannounced, only to be chastised by Dad.

'Please don't bring mad people into our house.'

'Why?' I asked

'Anything could happen. '

Dad was alarmed and while I did see his point, I also felt that was all part of the fun.

Introducing unwell friends to well friends could be amusing, especially if they didn't know what to expect. An old school friend of mine Rad met Bob, who quickly tried to impress Rad with his life story. He told Rad that he was expecting an MBE imminently, for services rendered to the Queen and that he used to be great friends with Princess Margaret. Rad looked baffled and didn't know what to say or how to react. He didn't know that Bob was an unwell, unemployed electrician. So, he just went with the flow. He asked Bob if he also knew the Queen in an informal capacity and whether she had thanked him personally for his services.

'Not half,' Bob replied

'What did she say?' asked Rad

'Bob, where would I be without you?'

'Crikey,' Rad replied.

Bob was now sensing an audience to his stories and was also sizing Rad up physically. Bob was thick-set, although had a disproportionately large belly.

I prompted Bob: 'Weren't you once interested in boxing, Bob?'

'Oh yes,' said Bob, 'If it wasn't for Henry Cooper, I would have been British Heavyweight Champion.'

Rad was now giggling and simply asked Bob if he was married or had any children.

'At one point or another, I have raised near on twenty children. The only one left is my stepson.' That last bit was true. Rad soon got the hang of being with my other friends and they liked him.

One sunny morning, I got a phone call out of the blue. It was Bob asking for a lift to a police station so that he could collect a rucksack handed in by one of his stepson's friends. I didn't know the full circumstances but agreed to take him. We arrived at the police station and Bob immediately addressed the Sergeant behind the desk.

'My stepson's rucksack has been handed in and I've come to collect it.'

'NAME?' the officer said sharply

'Who, mine or his?'

'Yours.'

'Bob..'

'Can you describe him?'

'Yes, he gets a bit lairy after a few drinks.'

We got there in the end. The policeman even came out to take my car registration for extra security, once he had reluctantly let Bob have the rucksack.

Bob had a girlfriend, Mildred, and they had met in hospital. She was also a colourful character and could be a smidgen off reality when it came to stories. Many years ago, she had worked at the BBC and purported to be an actress, although Bob didn't believe her. Once while we were chatting, she announced some interesting news.

'I went for a job at the BBC today.'

'How did you get on?' Bob said

'I was pipped to the post.'

'Who by?'

'Judy Dench.'

Chapter 10

Rupert

I first met Rupert in Southview Villa in Longrove Hospital, Epsom, in 1980. I will have been eighteen and this was my first breakdown. Rupert was in his early twenties. It was the first of many admissions and sections that we had together, over about twenty years. On this occasion, we'd both been sectioned for six months.

We immediately became friends and there was a mischievous side to him that I liked. During one of our first meetings, we were both in our pyjamas and Rupert persuaded me to leave the ward and run around the grounds. Soon we were running around a field, over and over again and despite my psychosis and confusion, I thought the whole thing was hilarious. After a while, I stopped and Rupert was still running around a field in his hospital dressing gown like his life depended on it.

Rupert was a sensitive man and it was reflected in his brilliant artwork, which he drew from his imagination. I thought he was a genius and I loved him very much. When he was outside hospital, he had an on /off relationship with a fiery Latin lady and he would bring gifts of his artwork to her, which he would just as quickly take away if he was upset with her. She'd be in the other room and in a flash, they'd be dismantled, and he'd be gone. On the other hand, he could also entertain her at his place, but that could prove tricky. Once, when she was dressed up and had arrived to see him, he panicked at the sound of her voice and immediately rang the Samaritans, while she waited patiently outside.

He was extremely protective of his work and if you called around to his house, you would be asked to wait outside while he hid, or rearranged his art, while you smiled at the notice on his door.

No leaflets or circulars ... Keep your rubbish to yourself.

During our stay in hospital, he told me a little about his difficult upbringing and we also shared humorous stories together. Sometimes we would go from the hospital into Epsom and when I had a visitor, we would all go into town. Sometimes this was with permission, sometimes not.

Another time, in one of the side rooms, I saw Rupert on his hands and knees at the feet of a stranger, taking the man's shoes off and putting them back on again. I could hear Rupert saying with the voice of a man in utter desperation,

'Oh no, I've got it wrong again.'

While the stranger, another patient, sat there motionless.

One evening, I was particularly unwell, and the 'heavy' nurses had surrounded me. I couldn't fight them, so I decided to do a spinning wheel movement with my arms, like a horizontal windmill, which I thought would be effective, and at that very moment Rupert opened the door and looked at me briefly, which gave me some hope, but no sooner was he there, then he was gone. The nurses jumped me, and I was given a forced injection. At that time, my illness was manifesting as grandiosity. If you were to ask me what I was thinking at these times or ask me what psychosis is, I would say it's a combination of confusion, grandiosity, panic, and paranoia. It is frightening in the moment and upsetting afterwards. You don't understand how or why you were so upset.

Rupert and I would still meet up outside the hospital and remain good friends. He told me that one day, a man in a Rolls Royce pulled up and asked him for directions and Rupert suggested he go along, as he was going there himself. He had no idea where the man was going but was enjoying the ride in such a posh car.

'Yes, left here,' he said," and a little bit further on,' and, 'perhaps go right there,' until the man finally chucked him out.

Rupert would regularly play cricket against one of his friends and they would meticulously keep score against each other. The grounds of the hospital would ring with cries such as:

'98 versus 72!'

'No, that last one didn't count!'

'Why?'

'I was in my pyjamas.'

Rupert had a particular style of his own and would wear a beaten-up old leather jacket and had a snazzy moustache and would bomb around the neighbourhood on his pushbike. Rupert was admitted to hospital forty-six times. Exactly half of those admissions were when he was on medication and the other half not.

He would sometimes ask me: 'What's the answer, women or religion?' and 'which is more important, my art, or my health?'

The answer to the second question turned out to be his art. He could draw quite brilliantly on the minimum amount of medication, but his health would suffer.

One evening, he threw himself off his balcony and left a big gap in the lives of all who knew and loved him.

Chapter 11
In and out

By the time I was in my early twenties, I had already been sectioned twice. It was decided that it was unhealthy for me to be living at home full time. So, I was moved into a halfway house for the vulnerable. A halfway house is a hostel for mentally ill people. You have a room in a block with a shared kitchen and bathroom, a common room and a garden. There you had to go to weekly meetings, which I hated. We used to have to say how you were doing and talk about short term and long-term plans. I was low and suffering from simmering feelings of anger, and I wanted to be at home. So, for a while, I used to sneak off on Friday afternoons for the weekend and go home. Generally, the staff turned a blind eye, but it was frowned upon. I would always dread the bus ride back on Sunday evenings.

I became friends with a man called Dick, who seemed to have his own agenda. He worked regularly but his only mental disability was his fear about his physical health. His mental health label was hypochondria.

Once a week, a patient was on dining duty. Your guest was invited into a small room with a cooker and a small table and chairs, and you would attempt to cook a meal for them while they patiently waited. The rules were always kept to and a staff member would pop their head round and check everything was okay. This was all in preparation for life on the outside. Your budget was one pound fifty and you had to present the receipt to the staff after shopping. It was always embarrassing asking for a receipt for a couple of baking potatoes. However, you were allowed to help yourself to spices from the kitchen.

When it was Dick's turn, he ordered us a takeaway pizza. Obviously, this blew the budget and made no use of the facilities. I just remember being delighted and laughing at Dick's subsequent argument with the staff.

After about a year, my social worker offered me alternative accommodation and I was relieved. Here, they wouldn't grill you at weekly meetings and that was a blessing. Even so, there were people with a mixture of vulnerabilities. Although it was run by a lady who kept us all on our toes. The main thing I remember about her was that she would often walk into a room and make a mild shriek:

'Eeahhh?!'

I never knew whether she was replying to, or asking a question. She had a good heart and I liked her and would sometimes walk her dog.

I began to become a little more confident and gradually some of my friends got back in touch. I also joined a cooking class and during this time, I met and fell in love with Mary. I moved in with her and this time it was a healthy setting, and we shared a flat in Cricklewood with an Irish crowd. Finally, I felt properly accepted. When people accept you, you don't feel the need to explain yourself and they see good things in you that you might not have seen yourself. You feel safe and because of that, your anxiety levels fall. I got a job as an Ambulance driver in a Jewish day centre and learnt a lot. The freedom of living life with healthy people was like a breath of fresh air.

I am now in my most recent accommodation, a flat in a block for vulnerable people, where I have been for twenty-five years. I have been broadly happy here; however, I have had the odd moment of confusion. I was recently driving into the close and an unwell woman that I remembered was standing at the bus stop just outside and she spotted me. I parked my car and walked towards the entrance to the building, and she suddenly appeared next to me.

'Sorry you can't come in,' I said.

I entered the building and began to walk up the stairs.

Rat tat tat tat: a loud noise came from the outside door that I had just closed.

Crikey, I thought. She's not giving up. I walked up the two flights of stairs and finally arrived at the door to my flat. I looked behind me nervously and entered. Two minutes later, the buzzer on the intercom sounded and I pressed to hear who it was.

'Yes," I said. 'Hello.'

'Postman.'

The voice had a strange high-pitched tone. I was worried it was the woman imitating the postman to try and get in.

I spoke through the intercom.

'Now you know you're not well. It's time you went back to mental hospital,' I replied.

'What?' the voice said. 'It's the postman.'

And it was.

Chapter 12
Mr 60s

I became friends with a man that I soon Nicknamed 'Mr 60s', because of the golden era that he had shone in the music business. He had been European representative for EM and also belonged to a band called Sun Dragon and had two top 50 hits.

Mr 60s had a great sense of humour, and he was bright, but seemed to be stuck in a groove, like one of his records.

'What happened to my wife?' he would say and, 'Why did I get divorced?' and 'What happened to my band?' and 'Where are my friends?'

Despite answering him as best you could, he couldn't get over the changes and the passage of time. I was fond of him and every now and again, we would go uptown to a music function and he would check on or collect royalties. Sometimes, I would visit him in a day centre and ask if he'd like to go out for a coffee.

One afternoon, bored after a couple of years of the usual questions, I replied to him, 'I know exactly where your wife is and I know exactly what she's doing.'

'Where is she?' he asked, eyes lighting up. 'What's she doing?'

'She's a petrol pump attendant in Carshalton.'

He laughed and laughed. A month or two later, Ian came bounding up to me with exciting news. 'Joe, I may have found a new girlfriend.'

'Great, what's she like?'

'She drinks too much; she smokes too much and she's not all there. She's ideal.'

Years passed and we had a lot of fun. We once pressed on Mick Jagger's intercom on Richmond Hill when he was still with Jerry Hall. I knew where he lived because Rupert, my artist friend, had sold him a couple of paintings

'Oh hi,' I said. 'I'm a friend of the artist, Rupert. Would you like to buy one of his paintings?'

'No thank you,' Jerry Hall said in her wonderful Texan drawl.

It was all a kind of mad nostalgia.

Mr 60s developed Motor Neuron disease near the end but still had the capacity to enjoy life and was very keen to receive visitors in the hospital. I used to bring along a motley crew of friends up to see him in the hospice in Watford. My sister, Lu, was situated on the way, so we'd stop off and visit. Although soon Lu and her husband asked me to stop visiting them on a Sunday!

At the time I thought, 'why? I'm equally nuts, and you can put up with me, so why not my friends?'

I didn't understand, but I respected their decision and stopped the double whammy visits. Now, many years later, I do understand that four of us calling in every week might have been a bit overwhelming.

One of the effects of Ian's Motor Neuron Disease was a weakness in his hands. One night, we were in the lounge area of the Intercontinental Hotel in Park Lane. We had asked for a cup of tea and they brought us an enormous silver teapot at a huge price and there was a harp playing. In a way, we were celebrating Ian's life. He was in his element and began talking loudly and full of pride.

'Yes, I was big in the sixties, 'he bragged, as he slid one finger into the handle of his china cup. 'European representative for EMI, two top fifty hits, and Joe ... could you get my finger out of this cup?'

Chapter 13

Plant man

My latest home was a flat within a housing block in Barnes which housed vulnerable people. I often wondered to myself, why is he or she vulnerable? Mostly, I would never know exactly, but may have got some idea once I'd got to know them.

One evening, I was walking down the stairs and a strange man began to climb up slowly towards me.

'Hello,' I said.

He mumbled something and shuffled past me. He was quite scary looking, a bit dishevelled with a scruffy beard and a walking stick. I bumped into him a few times over the next few weeks, and I began to warm to my scruffy neighbour. He would tend to his plants that he placed on each level down the stairs, and I nicknamed him 'Plant man.'

However, conversations were difficult and quite often, he would look completely past me and talk in a barely audible tone. In fact, if he did stop to chat, he was always physically turned at least ninety degrees away from my gaze. It was like he had made friends with the wall. Not only that, but we were also often on the move. I'd see him disappearing into his flat in mid conversation. This chat on the move was reciprocated. I too would sometimes enter my flat, which was next door to his, while we were talking. I would be halfway through saying goodbye when his door would shut.

He had a good work ethic and despite not having a regular job or boss, he would invent jobs for himself around the neighbourhood. He may do some gardening outside the local church or paint the railings surrounding the reservoir. Nobody would stop him, as he was no harm and he wasn't really breaking any rules.

One morning, I looked outside my window and saw three elderly ladies standing by the bus stop, on the pavement, next to the railings. I then noticed a hand holding a paintbrush poking through the railings, coming from the reservoir. Plant man was on the other side and completely camouflaged by the bushes. The ladies were very startled by the sight of this hand-held brush suspended amongst them and he had now created mild hysteria.

Another neighbour, Jim from downstairs, and I would sometimes have a bit of a chat.

'Have you seen plant man?' I would ask.

'He must have made good progress,' Jim would reply. 'Last thing I heard; he was painting Hammersmith Bridge.'

Another time, Jim might gossip: 'Did you hear, he was stopped by the police last night?'

'What for?'

'He was pushing a lawn mower and had a guitar under his arm, at one in the morning. Yeah, and he was quite annoyed he'd been stopped at all.'

'What was he doing with a lawnmower?'

'Someone said he was trying to grow a lawn in his flat.'

I mostly turned a blind eye to Plant man's eccentricities, but occasionally I would have to intervene, for example when another neighbour Ian was having a difficult time. He was short of money as he had given most of it away to charities in the hope it would guarantee his place in heaven.

On this occasion, Ian's shortage of money required drastic action. He began to knock on each of his neighbours' doors asking for money. He made it up as far as the plant man, who answered the door.

'Have you got a fiver?' Ian asked

'No.' Was the response.

There was a brief pause while Ian collected himself.

'Call yourself a Christian?' And he threw a punch .

Within seconds, they were wrestling and on the floor. A pot plant had been dislodged and Dave's walking stick was amongst them. I came out to intervene, but they were in gridlock and were not about to be separated.

I said, 'If you don't pack it in, I'm going to call the police.' And they didn't. So, moments later, I was on the phone to the police.

'Hello, yes, I want to report an ongoing fight.'

'Are there any weapons being used?'

'Yes, a walking stick and a pot plant.'

Life continued and I would sometimes see Plant man tending to his goldfish on the landing and things seemed to be back to normal in the block. Until one day I heard voices just outside my flat and went to investigate. There was a large man, who looked official, talking to Plant man.

'I am sorry to inform you that because of fire regulations we are going to have to remove everything blocking the stairs.'

This of course meant the plants and the goldfish. He was distraught and began waving his stick around.

'Please keep that stick away from me,' the man said.

At this point, I decided to try and distract plant man...

'Look at me,' I said. He turned around. 'What do I want to look at you for?

It seemed to work. In the end, the man told him that he was going to put it in writing and left. I knew that the trust meant business and soon enough, there were men in the building, and they began to clear the passageways of all his plants etc.

I felt sad for him, but I hadn't heard the last of the episode. I wasn't there when his stuff was taken out, but according to Jim, Plant man placed a flying Kung Fu kick at the last man, taking out the last plant. All he wanted was to tend his plants and look after his goldfish and do his made-up jobs but this interference had all become too much for him. He sadly had to have a spell in a psychiatric ward. I missed him, but in the circumstances, felt it may have been the best thing and looked forward to his safe return. He did come back two months later but the plants never returned to the stairwell.

Chapter 14

Pippa

I was visiting a friend in a psychiatric hospital in Epsom, when I noticed a pretty woman. She had striking blue eyes, shoulder-length hair and an alluring mixture of both classic and hippy dress sense. I went up to her and we chatted briefly and then I asked her name.

'Pippa,' she said.

'Hi, I'm Joe, can I get you a coffee?'

'Yeah sure, actually I can get you one from the kitchen,' she said.

I wasn't sure where the kitchen was, but she left and that was all I saw of her during my visit. However, she left an impression on me and I wondered if I would see her again.

Many months later, we bumped into each other. This time though, I was luckier, and we joked about our first meeting. We were in the opening lounge of a day centre and she offered me a coffee and this time promised to return.

She shortly reappeared with two china cups.

'Perfect,' I thought, 'I'm going to enjoy coming here.' I think by then I had drunk a lot of tea and coffee from plastic cups.

Pippa had a form of bi-polar disorder and later told me that she'd delayed being discharged from the centre since I'd arrived. So, we both had something to look forward to.

It was the beginning of an 'on, off' relationship that would last over twenty-five years. We were never in hospital together – I found out very recently that we were not allowed in the same place, although we would often visit each other, even if we weren't allowed in. One time, I had just won a few quid on a table tennis match whilst inside and Pippa was at the locked entrance door. I passed the cash under the door to Pippa, so that her visit wasn't totally fruitless. It was anyone's guess who was looking after who. It really was 'the blind leading the blind.'

We often took off together, despite who was on section (which means detained without your consent for your own safety). One night, we found ourselves on the run in Kingston and ended up in a bed and breakfast. At four in the morning, Pippa said she'd like a coffee and a ciggy. So, I went out on a mission. I came back half an hour later, with two ciggies and two cups of coffee.

At some point, I proposed to Pippa and gave her an engagement ring. It didn't last long, as during, or rather after a big argument, she smashed it to pieces with a hammer.

I began to call around to her house and if she wasn't in, I would leave my shoes and socks on the doorstep. Her Mum, Madge, used to think that was my calling card. Once, when Madge opened the door, I noticed her shoes and I was convinced that she had invested wisely in special ones for her daughter's marriage to me. I later found out that they were only a pair of carpet slippers. I also found Pippa's daughter's wig – I have no idea why her teenage daughter had a wig – Sometimes, I would wear it around the neighbourhood. I was never any good at keeping a low profile and so evading the police was always a problem.

Once they traced me back to Pippa's and after a struggle, I was handcuffed and led out into a van and taken back to hospital. Despite the use of force, I found the police were always fair with me and spoke to me with kindness. When you're on section, the police have the right to bring you back to hospital by whatever means. I didn't like being cuffed behind my back but once I was in the van, I knew I was on my way back to safety. Also, I liked the sirens – when you're high in your mania, you enjoy the drama.

That time, I was quite baffled as to why I was being taken away and had even borrowed Madge's phone the previous night to ring my local priest at four am, to check on arrangements for mine and Pippa's special day. We were never getting married; there was no wedding; this had become my confused fantasy.

And so, the merry go round continued. Pippa was now in Queen Mary's hospital, and I was determined to visit her. This time, cross country. I was trying to avoid the police but was getting into a fine mess. I crossed a brook and had mud up to my knees and had somehow come upon a pineapple. My shoes had long gone, and I was in a bit of a state. I finally reached the ward and pressed the buzzer. The nurse came out and I told her who I had come to see. The pineapple was accepted, but I wasn't.

When Pippa was free, we would be running around, off our crazy heads – not on drugs, just on our natural manic highs. Neither knew what we were doing, but we were enjoying each other's company, like a pair of love-struck, headless chickens.

I took her out to a restaurant, thinking I had booked it, but when we arrived there was no record of the booking, and the restaurant was full. I immediately hailed a taxi which was close by. We got in and after a short distance, probably sixty yards, I asked if we could stop. Pippa got out and so did I, after a look from the driver.

'Did you pay?' Pippa asked me.

'It's ok, it's sorted.' I thought the driver's wink was one of acceptance, as if to say *This one's on me*.

I couldn't have been further from the truth. He got out of his cab and came tearing after me, fuming.

'What are you playing at?'

I didn't say anything but started to imitate the look he had given me in the cab, so I began winking at him.

'What are you winking at, you moron? I want four pounds.'

I tried to exaggerate my winking, to emphasise the almost coded, special look he had given me, but now Pippa had spotted the problem, and after separating her winking boyfriend from the irate cab driver, she paid him and there was no more fuss.

We are still great friends. Although we never did get married. Pippa had young children when we met, who are now grown up. I have a teenage son with another woman. I will always remember those chaotic times together. Even to this day, she is the best person to talk to when I'm feeling ill. She is funny, much funnier than she realises, and she knows me and understands a lot about mental illness.

We're both on the phone to each other regularly. Sometimes she will phone and tell me she's had the most terrible week but when I ask her about it, reply that she doesn't want to talk about it.

Or she might phone me first thing in the morning and say: 'How are you, Joe?'

'Fine thanks,' I respond. 'And you?'

'Not bad, I'll speak to you later.

The phone call would end, then twenty minutes later, she would call again as if we hadn't spoken and say: 'Hi, it's me, how are you?'

And I would reply: 'The same as I was twenty minutes ago.'

Chapter 15

Ian Powell

About fifteen years ago, I was living in the sheltered accommodation where I live now and I was surprised by a knock at the door. It was eight o'clock in the evening. It was my new neighbour Ian and he wanted to borrow a tie. I soon realised that he was an extraordinary character. He was a middle-aged man and he had just begun a paper round and had also started acting in the local amateur dramatics. He had always had a fascination with radio and soon had his sights on becoming a hospital radio DJ . But in the meantime, he would be regularly ringing up radio stations with live banter. He even rang up a children's Christmas show and was asked by Tony Blackburn how old he was.

Ian replied, 'Forty-six!'

Soon he was writing all sorts of scripts and managed to get a written reply from Chris Tarrant, who teased him about his lack of talent.

'Ah,' Ian said. 'Competition at last! '

He had also written a James Bond film script and, when made into a film, he was going to play a character called Dick Leno, a San Francisco DJ. I popped in to see Ian one morning and he said

'Joe, I've made a recording of part of my James Bond movie. Would you like to hear it?'

'Yes, I'd love to.' I sat in anticipation.

'So, James,' came the voice out of the tape recorder. 'The tape has fallen into the wrong hands. What is MI5 going to think about that?'

Another voice – but still Ian said: 'Get out!'

It made no sense whatsoever . I laughed inwardly, as I had learnt not to correct him. Although I often felt that I should. It was as if he were in a permanent manic phase, and he certainly wouldn't listen to criticism.

He began sending scripts all over the place and had plans to have his own chat show called 'Powell's People.' I think this might have come from Pan's People, the popular dance group from Top of the Pops.

'Ian,' I said, humouring him. ``Would there be any room for me on one of your shows?'

'Yes,' he said. 'You could sweep up.'

His religious fanaticism continued, and he would always tell me God was looking after him. One night, he left his home to get a packet of cigars from the local petrol station in Mortlake and ended up on the M1. He told me afterwards,

'God answered my prayers.'

'How?' I asked.

'I was kneeling down on the hard shoulder of the motorway praying and the police came and picked me up!'

Chapter 16
The fishing trip

Rev was a nickname my mate Dick had earned not from the clergy but during his biking days. He was someone I had met in a halfway house, and we immediately hit it off and became friends. He preferred me to call him Dick. I liked that because it felt more exclusive. He called me Joe. His illness was unusual, if not unique, and it was a genuine illness eighty percent of the time. The other twenty percent, he was using to his advantage, depending on the situation. He suffered from hypochondria, with a splash of paranoia thrown in.

It first came to my attention when I noticed an array of helping aids he would use. For example, a walking stick, a hearing aid and his notorious neck brace. I thought it was all quite odd and funny. One of the women in the hostel had asked him to go out with her and he told her quite frankly, that he couldn't, on the grounds that he was dying. There was always some new and complicated illness that he was suffering from, although five minutes before closing time in my local pub, he could do the two hundred yards sprint to get last orders in the next pub, at an illness-defying speed.

Once, when we were out and about, I noticed him staring down towards the floor with a look of shock. I picked up the object of concern and asked him what was wrong. The object was nothing more sinister than a rolled cigarette that had fallen from behind his ear.

'Thank God for that,' he said.' I thought a bit of me ear had just dropped off.'

We arranged to go on a fishing trip to Hampton Court. We arrived as early as we could at the local fishing tackle shop and he confidently chatted to the owner and bought some fishing tackle (neck brace firmly in place). As we headed towards the river, Dick mentioned a doctor's appointment he had in the afternoon, so I agreed to lend him the car. At the river, we relaxed and fished and soon enough, he caught an impressive three-pound trout. While he was basking in his catch, I reminded him of his appointment. Off he went with my car keys in hand and neck brace firmly on.

When he arrived, he told me later, he was concerned by the presence of a second doctor, which unsettled him . On the way back from the doctor's, Dick went via the fishing tackle shop to tell the guy there about the catch, this time without his neck brace. The first thing the man said to Dick was,

'You're having a scam, aren't you mate?'

Obviously, the man didn't understand Dick's mental illness.

Dick made his way back to me, looking worried. I asked him what was wrong, and he replied

'I think the doctors have been onto the fishing tackle shop.'

Chapter 17
Mixed nuts

Ned and I were often locked up together on the same wards. It was almost like a revolving door for us. On the outside, I had a weakness for drink, especially when I was getting my bipolar high and Ned had a weakness for drink and drugs, which always landed him in hospital sooner or later.

We were friends. When one of my well friends came to visit me in hospital, Ned might be sitting on a couch in the hospital lounge, smoking a ciggy.

'Oh, hi,' he would say, as if he was in his own front room. 'Joe's just in the other room.'

We had a lot of good times together, but it wasn't all fun and games. Both of us lost years of freedom, being over-medicated and having forced injections at times for our unpredictable illnesses and rebellious tendencies.

He had met my ex-girlfriend Mary often and had also come to the funeral of my fiancée, Julie, who died of a drug overdose. Julie is a whole other story – a passionate affair in which I was tempted to take drugs along with her but didn't. It was so intense that at times it felt like one of us dying was inevitable, it was just a question of who. Fortunately, I eventually learnt to take safer decisions for my health. Julie never got that far.

But back to Ned, who would also come up and visit our mutual friend Mr 60's in the hospice when he was dying. So, there was plenty of shared history outside the hospitals as well.

One time, when we were in hospital in Tolworth, we were allowed out for a couple of hours. Coincidentally, the eclipse of the sun was also about to happen. There was great anticipation among some of the patients. A woman patient who had been hanging around decided to tag along.

I asked Ned, 'Will she be ok?'

He said, 'oh she'll be alright.'

So, when the cab arrived, we all jumped in. I asked to go to Surbiton and was chuffed that we were going to see the eclipse in time. We arrived and soon enough, a crowd had gathered. It was getting darker by the second as the moon was eclipsing the sun; 'going, going,' the crowd started to chant and then slightly before the total eclipse, our new friend got over excited and screamed

'It's gone.'

And simultaneously threw her handbag miles into the air. The spectacle was magnificent and so was the eclipse. Momentarily we were in darkness. Finally, when we managed to retrieve her handbag, we returned to the hospital safely.

More recently, Ned would pass the time of day, hanging around outside the Richmond Royal Hospital with Lawrence, my friend from the day centre. Ned and Lawrence weren't exactly friends but would tolerate each other.

Over the years, during hospital stays, I had also got to know Lawrence and I always warmed to him. He was a bit like a sad clown. He had a funny way of walking. It was like he was being pulled along like a puppet on a string. You could never tell quite where the next foot was going, and his upper body had a weird way of almost not connecting to his legs. Lawrence had always thought I was a policeman, or rather he said he did. So, I would play along with it. If he managed to get to my place without incident, I would cook him a meal. We would be relaxing, chatting and I might offer him a cup of tea. When I was in the kitchen, I would lean over, just out of sight and speak into an imaginary intercom connected to an imaginary police station.

'So far, so good,' I would say. I would then turn to Lawrence and ask, 'White with one sugar?'

'Yes please,' he would answer, with a look of bewilderment.

Later, after we had been chatting for a while, I would leap up and go back into the kitchen and speak into the intercom again: 'That won't be necessary at this stage.'

I'm not sure he believed me because he was so funny and clever. I think he was just playing along for his own fun.

I had known Colin for what seemed like ages. We had gone to the same-day centres and rehabilitation venues, and he was a familiar face.

He was well known for his depressing look on life and his favourite expression was,

'Cursed be the day I was born.'

Coincidently, that was the same expression as the long-suffering Job in the Bible. Job is also my middle name.

Trying to cheer Colin up was a lost cause. I might go for a drink with him, and he would be nursing a pint and say,

'This will be the death of me.' Or 'It's taken me twenty-five years to discover the damage that drink's been doing to my body.'

I remember telling that to my Mum and she said, 'That seems an awfully long time.'

Over a period of years, Colin and I had gone for long walks, played golf together, discussed the meaning of life and he had even helped decorate my flat, during which he downed strong lagers and assured me he could still decorate to a high standard, even while drinking.

'Joe, these strong lagers have very little effect on me. I'm totally used to them. They're like shandy to me.'

As he was finishing his sentence, he wobbled slightly and held onto the sink to steady himself. On another occasion, we had gone for a drink and arrived at a busy pub and ended up at a table smack in the middle of the room. Colin began to lecture me on the sensitivities of the feet and what he had learnt through a medical examination. He then took one shoe and sock off and briefly explained the various acupoints on the foot, before plonking his foot on the table, much to my shock and the rest of the pub's. He touched one part of his foot and let out an agonisingly loud cry and, with his face contorted, screamed

AAAAAAUUUGGGGHHHHH!

With a sense of relief to both me and everyone in the pub, he brought his foot down and put his shoe and sock back on.

I suggested that I might try, and Colin said

'No, it's far too dangerous.'

Funnily enough, Colin never had psychosis, he just had chronic depression and was incredibly eccentric.

Chapter 18
We're from the other side

During my period of less severe illness, I was able to drive and owned a car. On one occasion, this was about twenty years ago, I decided to take my four friends to Hyde Park: Lawrence, Ian Powell, Mr Sixties and Ned, and I think this story shows how difficult it is to organise an outing with people, all of whom suffer from varying degrees of poor mental health.

We were all in a jolly mood when we met. Lawrence had managed to find himself in the front seat, which raised an eyebrow or two from Ian and Mr Sixties, although Ned didn't bat an eyelid, as he was bang in the middle at the back and he liked that spot.

I had decided that I had to be in control, as we all had a history of mental illness and I was driving. I felt responsible for any mishaps or misdemeanours.

Within minutes, Ned tried to cadge a fag off Ian Powell and Ian suggested Mr Sixties could help, as he clearly had more baccy than him. Mr Sixties looked upset and said, 'Don't you ever keep your own baccy?'

'Oh, come on Sixties, it's only one roll-up,' said Ned and Mr Sixties reluctantly agreed, passing Ned a Rizla paper and a small amount of tobacco.

Lawrence was unusually quiet and was wearing a pair of dark shades. Every now and then, he gave a funny smile and said, 'lovely.'

Meanwhile, Ian was happily tapping a tune on his lap and offering pieces of croissant to everyone and halfway into the journey asked if we could stop and pick up some more baccy and a takeaway coffee.

At that point, I said' maybe it's better to wait until we get to the park.'

When we arrived, Mr Sixties immediately became very sensitive and paranoid...

'Was that bloke just staring at me?' he said. 'What about him? He's looking at me funny.'

But it was his own paranoid stares that were the main reason people were looking back at him and that was exacerbating the problem. To make matters worse, Ned had just asked him for another roll-up. Mr Sixties stormed off and soon we were all trying to catch up with him. Especially me. As the group leader, I didn't want to lose any of them.

Somehow, we arrived at a café and we took our takeaway coffees and found a nice piece of grass to sit down on. Lawrence was looking particularly strange. He had a large overcoat on, a large camera perched around his tummy, the straps hanging round his neck and two gardening gloves, one poking out from each pocket. I then spotted two policemen coming towards us. They stopped right next to us.

'Where are you lot from then?' one of them said.

Lawrence turned around slowly and said, 'We are from the other side.'

The policeman persisted, 'That sounds a bit funny, mate. What do you mean?'

I perked up and felt strangely authoritative, 'We're alright, just enjoying the park.'

Like a magic wand, they turned around and left us.

We enjoyed the rest of our time in the park and soon we were back in the car and on our way. Ian, tapping on his coffee cup, Lawrence looking menacing in shades, Ned, finally with fags and Mr Sixties relaxing and laughing loudly at my bad jokes.

Chapter 19

Bob save the Queen

Another mate from one of the day centres was Bob, who believed he had foiled a terrorist threat at Heathrow airport in the late seventies. He reckoned he had diffused a bomb while working there as an electrician. He is awaiting his knighthood.

Years later, there was another threat, this time more serious; the whole of London was in danger. He felt it, he told me, *in his water*.

Bob would often chat to his friend Rodney, a simple man who would often come over for a cup of tea first thing in the morning. They would tell each other stories about their earlier lives. Bob would tell Rodney how he had left home early to join the merchant navy and Rodney laid claim to having served in the Royal Navy. Bob didn't believe him, though he never told him directly.

On one of these mornings, Bob was feeling strongly about the threat to London, and to the Queen in particular, and felt the need to take the trip up to the Chelsea Barracks to warn her. He told Rodney he would go immediately but was short of cash.

'Rodney,' he said.

'Lend us a fiver, will you? I must go and save the Queen.'

Rodney agreed and Bob went on his mission, the journey was nothing compared to the vital message he needed to pass on.

When he got back, he told Rodney the whole story. Once there, he marched up to a soldier and said, 'I'd like to speak to the adjutant.'

The adjutant duly arrived, responding quickly enough to his message, Bob felt. Then Bob spoke out in a commanding voice: 'I have some very important news to pass on to the Queen.'

'Yes of course,' replied the adjutant. 'Can I have your name sir?'

'The name is Bob, but let's move on to more urgent matters.' Bob was now feeling a very real sense of importance and was also impatient due to the urgency of the situation.

'Buckingham Palace,' he said, 'and the whole of London is in imminent danger. There is a risk of a bomb.'

'Thank you, Bob,' said the adjutant, 'You are a fine man. I shall pass the message on. '

'What happened next?' Rodney asked, amazed.

' Well,' Bob said. 'She was out the side gate of Buckingham palace and onto her souped-up gold-plated Yamaha 50cc, over Chertsey Bridge and down the Staines Road before the emergency services could keep up with her.'

' Crikey,' said Rodney. 'Did she get a chance to put her crash helmet on?'

Bob looked aghast.

'Are you joking? We're talking about the Queen here! Nothing but the best and that includes her crown!'

Finally, she arrived at Windsor Castle and into relative safety, where Bob was of course awaiting her arrival.

'She must have been very grateful,' Rodney said. 'What did she say?'

'Bob,' 'I don't know how you do it.'

'I expect she was in a state of shock when she arrived. Did she have a roll-up and a stiff drink?'

Bob puffed out his chest indignantly.

'The Queen doesn't smoke roll-ups! She's on twenty Lambert and Butler a day!'

'Bob,' Rodney said. 'You're a great man.'

'Thank you,' Bob replied.

Chapter 20
The visitor (1990)

For anyone with serious mental health difficulties, money is an issue. I have worked in many jobs but have always been too ill to hold them down and have had to stop. As a very young man I lived here and there and it wasn't until I was twenty-eight years old that I came to where I live now, a specially designed block for vulnerable people, where I have been for thirty years, and where I have been able to become well enough to live without crisis. A stable home has helped hugely, in addition to the birth of my son, which made the biggest difference of all. At my sheltered accommodation, the rent is low. I have some benefits, which allow me to survive, but have been lucky enough to get a little extra help from charities, without which life would be very difficult.

Before I had any extra help, my social worker, Janet, came up with a solution to my shortage of money. This will have been about thirty years ago, around the time I moved into the sheltered block.

'There's a charity specialising in helping people with your background, who are down on their luck,' she said.

' My background, what do you mean?'

'Well, it's for vulnerable, well-to-do people.'

She meant middle-class. I had never been described like that before, but I thought I'd go along with it anyway.

' They would probably visit you at your home first,' she said.

'OK.'

The first visit was arranged, and a smartly dressed man arrived. I told him a bit about myself.

'I can tell you've had a difficult time,' he interrupted. 'But what about your family background?' 'Oh, well,' I said. 'My grandmother was a debutante.'

'My, my, a deb!

'And my father had some important connection in Burma.'

'Really?'

'Yes, well, I know he was conceived halfway up the Irrawaddy'

He gave me a funny look. Nevertheless, I was accepted. From then on, once a week, a payment was made into my account, and I was visited regularly by people from the organisation to ensure my circumstances hadn't changed. This went on for twenty years or so – I had my son during this time - until I was informed that the charity was cutting down on financial support and that my next visit might well be my last.

I made it my mission to make a big effort. I cleaned my curtains, mopped the floors, and I did the washing up particularly well. But it all seemed a bit dishevelled - my cooker and fridge shared over thirty years between them and were looking a bit past it.

Recently, my uncle had sent me a birthday photo of Ian Fleming smoking a ciggy with a fancy cigarette holder, so I put that in prime position. One of my goldfish had died since the last visit and, as the visitor had remarked how pretty they both were, I camouflaged the surviving one with extra greenery, hoping to disguise the fact that one of them had died. Photos were put into position and even my African artefacts were placed in view. That should impress them, I thought.

So, the time had come, and I was nervous. When the lady from Elizabeth Finn Care arrived, I hovered over my photos, hoping she would notice them, and then we sat down. I offered her a cup of tea.

'No, thank you.'

'Do you mind if I have one?'

I began to raise myself out of the chair to put the kettle on.

'If you really want one.'

I was in Limbo, neither standing nor sitting.

'No, I'll be fine,' I said, and fell back into the chair.

When there was a lull in the conversation, I leapt up like a surprised frog and took the photo display off the wall and brought it over for her to look at . I proudly showed her photos of my family and even some of my parents meeting famous people and some of which I was especially proud of, like the ones of my son growing up. We continued our conversation and then we were abruptly interrupted by a knock at the door. I went and opened it slightly.

It was Maria, an old flame. She was a fiery and pretty loopy Latin American woman that I had known for many years.

'Are you entertaining?' she asked, peering over my shoulder to try and get a look.

'Well, actually I've got a visitor.'

'We could come to some kind of arrangement,' she persisted, sounding like a strange, foreign military officer. I chose to ignore her comments – sometimes conversations between two people, both of whom are unwell, can be difficult to decipher - and even I had no idea what she was on about. I firmly closed the door, went back to my visitor, and apologised for the interruption. I then heard another noise that sounded like the opening of my letterbox, followed by a strong vocal burst from Maria.

'I've met gipsies like you before,' she shouted and then there was silence.

My visitor simply asked me for a glass of water and muttered, 'Friend?'

I smiled. But I was also hoping she hadn't heard all of Maria's remarks. We didn't talk about anything in particular after that. She might have asked about my family and my health and I would also have asked about her family. When she told me she had to leave, I was relieved, but also sad, as I knew it may be the last time she visited me and the last time they could help financially.

And it was. After that, they gradually reduced my payments until they stopped altogether. It was a blow, but I just about survived until another charity offered to help and give me a similar amount – about twenty pounds a week – which makes a great difference to me. It might seem expensive, supporting mentally ill people week by week, but I have known many people in this situation as well as myself. I know that the consequences of not giving support in this way would result in much more expensive, not to mention much more upsetting treatment in hospital.

Chapter 21
The metal gate, the ring and the funeral (around 2000 – last hospital stay)

Around 2000, I was about thirty-eight, I was being kept at P1, the psychiatric ward in Queen Mary's hospital in Roehampton. Although on a section, I was allowed out occasionally with permission. This time, I didn't escape, but I did wander down to the nearest pub. I must have had a little money; I know that if you stayed inside for less than six weeks, they didn't stop your benefits. Hours later, I staggered back to the hospital and found myself locked out of the grounds itself. But in my state, I didn't notice that I could have got in via the main entrance, a hundred yards or so ahead, which was open.

In front of me was an imposing gate and I felt that the only way in was over it. The gate had spikes on the top. It was like breaking out of prison only to break back in. I stepped onto a ledge and managed to put one leg into a hole and raise myself up. Then the same with the other. So far so good. I lifted the other leading leg over the top. I was now perched right above the spikes, straddled with one leg either side and taking the strain of my body weight on both arms.

Then I tried to swing the roadside leg over the spikes to join the other, on the hospital side, but I couldn't quite get my leg over.

'Crikey,' I shouted.

I had caught a spike. It had gone through my trousers and just missed my particulars.

I was impaled. What now?

There was almost no room for manoeuvre. The spike had a barb, like a fishing hook and my forearms were tiring. With a final burst of strength, I lifted my body up and off the spike and flung my leg up and over and was free.

Sometimes, mental illness means that you let down those you love, and that can be very hard. Around this time – as with many of my life's events, I can't remember clearly when - my brother Tim was about to get married to a lovely local woman called Leanne and our family had been invited to Australia for the Wedding. But best of all, for me, Tim had invited me to be his best man. Apart from the speech and the proceedings for the big day, there was a small matter of the ring to worry about.

I was honoured to be asked to be best man and normally I love to do a bit of showing off to family and friends. This time, however, it was to a relatively new and large crowd that I wasn't familiar with and my anxiety had already begun on the plane journey to Australia. On top of my usual travelling nerves, there was the best man speech to think about, which was exacerbating my anxiety.

The whole family had gone for the wedding and my sister Bex with all good intentions, had begun to coach me, even after we had arrived. The more she tried to help, the more nervous I became. Despite my determination, I was beginning to crack under the pressure. My reputation had preceded me. For many years and for patches of time, I may have appeared fearless, even to Tim and now I was a nervous wreck.

In the end, my sister Lu walked in to find me crying with stress and consoled me. My family realised the speech was too much for me. Dad stepped in and, on the day, made a very funny speech which turned out to be fantastic, and which was a big relief for me.

Meanwhile, Leanne's Uncle had agreed to marry the happy couple. His name was Wally and he was a priest and dearly loved by all who knew him. Tim, Wally and I practised the ceremony together to iron out any problems with the ring.

'Where do I stand?" said Tim – we were in the living room at the time.

'How close should I be?' I added, 'When do I pass the ring to Tim?' Wally was very calm and kept reassuring both of us.

'Everything is ok. Come the big day, it will run like clockwork,' he said, smiling confidently at the two of us.

The big day did come and when I passed the ring to Tim, it dropped on the altar floor and Uncle Wally stepped on it. We laughed about that – sometimes when things happen in the moment, it's easier. It's thinking about things going wrong that's the worst.

Anxiety is made up of so many things. I get scared of making a fool of myself, appearing to be mentally ill, security guards and authority figures are triggering because they remind me of hospitals. Travelling is stressful for those who suffer from anxiety because it feeds on the unknown. If you travel far away, there are so many stages at which something can go wrong – you might miss the flight, you might not be able to find your way to the right place, I would feel self-conscious sitting next to a stranger, worried I might not be able to make the right kind of conversation – for example, the question, what do you do for a living? is one I would find difficult because my work is often voluntary.

So, on visits to Australia, on my way to see Tim, I would find the trips quite stressful. But when I was finally through customs and I would see Tim in arrivals, suddenly, like a cool mountain breeze, my worries would be blown gently away to be replaced by a feeling of joy. I can remember one time seeing him there.

'Joe,' he called out and I was greeted with a big bear hug. We went straight to his car and I lit up a cigarette and smoked with relief. We had just got out of the airport, when Tim said,

'Patrick died.'

I said, 'Who is he?'

'Jenny's husband.'

'Who is she?'

'Never mind, have you got something smart to wear? The funeral's tomorrow. And by the way, we're going to be pallbearers.'

It seemed a bit strange that I was going to be a pallbearer on my second day in Oz, without even knowing the deceased, but I decided to go with the flow.

Wally – the priest - visited the house where Patrick had died and talked to his best friend, David, about the circumstances of his death.

'It all happened so soon, Wal,' said David. 'We were having a good drink. Probably twenty pints or so and he just keeled over.'

'Good God,' said Wally. 'Yeah, it must have been a dirty glass.'

The day of the funeral arrived and as usual, Tim and I were fussing over the proceedings: where to stand, how heavy was the coffin and which side of the grave would we go? And we both worried about the technique for lowering the coffin into the ground. It took me back to childhood and responsibilities in church when we were altar boys.

The hearse arrived and there was a gathering of mourners milling around the grave. Initially, four men, including me and Tim, picked up the coffin. I peered over at Tim and he was looking serious. We approached the grave. The weight of the coffin, the uneven ground and the loose gravel surrounding the grave caused me to lose my footing and my balance and I fell in. This caused a huge tilt to the angle of the coffin and at one point both me and half the coffin were in the hole together.

'Tim, help 'I cried out

I managed to clamber back up, with the help of a strong grasp from Tim's hand and I also managed to regain my composure and, this time, all went well. I apologised to the funeral goers and particularly to Jenny.

Chapter 22
The stranger 2010

By now I'd had my son Daniel and he would have been about eight. I often found myself with half an hour to spare, before picking him up and would go and sit in a small complex by the river and have a coffee to while away that time. It was always relatively empty there and I felt no pressure. Even the underground car park had free parking for one hour. There was a cinema, bar and restaurant and I was happy to be there, until it was necessary to leave. On this occasion, I noticed an elderly man of Indian-looking descent, sipping a Guinness at a small table, near the exit to the balcony.

I passed his table and went onto the balcony where I could smoke and admire the natural beauty of the river. I watched the boats go by and the stationary ones rocking and tilting in the breeze and even the occasional swirl, as a large fish would pluck an insect off the top.

The man began to light his pipe. He had an air of dignity and presence. He was smartly dressed and wore a pencil-thin moustache, which added to his gentlemanly demeanour. The sun was low, but bright for this time of year and in places, it lit up the river beautifully. After a brief silence, I decided to chat to him.

'We're lucky with the weather,' I said.

'No, we bloody are not, those bloody bastards get everywhere. I've had it up to here with them. It's like the middle of winter and you won't find anything here.'

The more he talked, the angrier he became, until I found myself a vessel for his ranting. I had no clue who these bastards he was referring to. The rant built to a crescendo and his eyes appeared to explode with fury, and I began to panic a little.

Had I done something to offend him, I wondered.

I started to smile and nod gently, putting my head a little to one side. I was trying to think of tolerant body movements to at least pacify him. I also became aware that he was now making very little sense and I became conscious of the time. So, I briefly made my excuses and left, wondering again what had caused this onslaught. I peered over my shoulder and noticed he had sat down again and was happily sipping his Guinness and reading his paper, on his table by the exit to the balcony.

I saw him again several times after and he would acknowledge me with a small wave or a nod of his head but if he ever started talking, he would go off on a torrent of nonsensical angry rubbish. All of which just goes to show that even when the outside is pristine and groomed, it doesn't necessarily follow that the inside is as neat and tidy. Mental illness has many forms.

Chapter 23

The river and the unicorn

I have always fished and often fish the River Wey in Ripley at dawn, because that's when the fish are feeding and the river is at its most beautiful. Often, whilst driving along the A3 to get to the fishing spot, it felt like a race against time and I would put my foot down on the accelerator to get there for sunrise.

This time, I needn't have worried about being late for dawn, as I had made a big error and I was an hour and a half early. What made matters worse, I had arrived in the pitch black and I was scared. I nearly turned the car around, to head home, but I dug my heels in. I felt very uncomfortable, sitting in the middle of nowhere, alone, in the middle of the night. I sat in this remote car park as quiet and still as death.

I thought I could hear noises from the bushes nearby and memories of a trip to Africa I'd made in my twenties returned. But there were no hippos or lions here. My senses seemed more acute. Just as I scanned the tree lined forest, barely visible through the darkness, I spotted a horse in the undergrowth, but more worrying, it had something poking from its forehead. I dismissed this vision in the night and decided it must have been a stray horse from the nearby fields, if indeed it was anything.

Eventually, I made my way to the river to set up for fishing, one eye on my fishing tackle and one over my shoulder. Soon I was ready. I cast my line into the river and almost simultaneously, I could hear the first bird, the very first one, in its dawn chorus and then a tug on the line.

'Thank God,' I thought to myself, as I started to play with the fish and the first rays of sunlight began to peep through the trees.

The river was covered in a beautiful blanket of mist. There were cows and horses in the nearby fields. It was just me and the river and I had just caught a fish in this magical place. Gone was the fear from the night. It was replaced by a feeling of peace and I savoured it.

Chapter 24
The Africa trip

In 1993, I was about thirty-three and was planning to meet my girlfriend Mary in Africa. She had gone out with her friend slightly earlier than me, as I planned to join her later, and was staying in a campsite.

Once in Kenya, and when I had arrived at the camp, I met an Aussie man who had set up his mini café on the beach. He told me where Mary's tent was. Although I couldn't see her, I was tired from the journey and decided to crash out in her tent.

We soon met and were delighted and made up for lost time. We decided to go on a boat excursion to a remote coral reef. Along the way, we were joined by a school of dolphins. They were diving and swimming next to the boat. Mary dived into the sea like it was second nature to her and I put on my goggles in trepidation and went in. I could see a group of dolphins underneath me in a circle. It was mesmerising and chilling, all at the same time.

We made our way back and settled into beach life for a while. However, an opportunity arose for me to join a safari full of Dutch travellers and I decided to go. Mary was happy for me. When we were leaving, I called out to her,

'Mary, have you got any matches?'

She ran up the beach and threw me a lighter, I caught it from the back of the truck, and I waved her goodbye. I soon made friends with the group. They all spoke immaculate English and were all quite tall.

On our first night, we pitched our tents just outside Nairobi and settled in. The next morning, from a long way off, we could see three Masai warriors coming towards us. Like the iconic scene in the desert from Laurence of Arabia. When they finally arrived, I asked them if I could take a photo. They seemed offended and left soon after. Later, our leader joked that it was my liver for breakfast.

I became worried and retreated to my tent. Soon, a man came over to check if I was okay. He was a peaceful-looking man with round glasses and slightly hippyish.

'Hey Joe, don't worry about the Masai, our leader was only joking. Will you be alright?'

'Yes fine, I'm just happy to be on my own for a while.'

But I wasn't, I was darned scared and paranoid, not a good combination in the middle of Africa.

'Why not try a Valium,' the guy said. 'They help me.'

And so, I did, and it helped.

Despite the strange circumstances, I warmed to him and felt a kindred spirit. His name was Luco.

That night, there was a thunderstorm, and my tent became flooded. So, I crawled out and climbed the steps of the truck and awoke our leader and we both shouted in shock. During the drama and in my fear, I had mistaken our driver for a waiting Masai, who I think was more frightened of me than I was of him. Soon, during the immense storm, one by one, everyone entered the truck, with a few swigs of brandy to nurse us through the night.

During the coming days, we passed Mount Kilimanjaro and were on our way to the Ngoro Gora crater. I saw lakes lit up with the pink cascade of thousands of flamingos. The energetic and funny ostriches running at full stretch next to the truck. We even saw the migration of the wildebeest, which would jump in startlement at our whooping. Aside from the migration was a small herd of wildebeest in a circle protecting their young, with two hyenas harassing them and a lone lion sitting patiently and lazily nearby. We travelled through the vast Serengeti, and I remember smiling to myself as a man cycled past from nowhere, as though he was off to the local shop. We even arrived at a lake full of hippos and one by one we stalked up to the water's edge and spied on them.

Meanwhile, my sister Lu and her husband Dave had also travelled to Africa. We weren't meant to be in the same country, but Dave had driven all day and at a certain point, got out of his Jeep and said to Lu:

'That bloke walks just like Joe'

And she shouted, 'It is Joe.'

We were all absolutely amazed to find ourselves in the same spot. I introduced them to my travelling group and they joined us. We toured the crater, seeing beautiful wildlife, but we didn't see the elephants. That night, we trucked it up a mountain path to a remote restaurant and had a few drinks. On the way back, I could make out two enormous rears belonging to elephants.

'Yes, sure,' someone said. 'Pink elephants.' They clearly didn't believe me, but I knew I'd seen elephants in the darkness.

We were now close to the camp and we got out of the truck. I called Luco to come and join me. Sure enough, there *were* two elephants but this time they were joined by an enormous male, with huge tusks and they were only about twenty-five yards away. Luco was short-sighted.

'It's not an elephant,' he said, peering at them. 'It's too big, is it a tree?'

Then it moved. There was a special moment between us; totally calm and totally peaceful. The elephants slowly turned away and returned to the bush and the man with the bow and arrow, guarding the camp, had fallen asleep at the bottom of a large tree.

Soon after, Luco and I left the safari and were on our own. We took a boat across Lake Victoria and arrived at a remote village. Our first greeting was from a witch doctor selling various potions. I had a slight hangover, so I pointed to my head and was given something to sniff and I promptly began to sneeze, which got the small crowd laughing. We moved on and the Dutch gang seemed a long way away.

We planned to go to Rwanda and managed to blag a very bumpy ride on a small truck, which went on for hours. The next day, Luco and I climbed a stagnant volcano in the rainforest with a guide. I couldn't keep up, so I climbed up a tree for protection and waited for them.

After a while, my mind wandered, and I began asking myself questions: what am I doing up this tree? How long should I stay here? and what if they can't find me on their way down?'

They were taking ages and I decided to climb down from the tree. I began walking down something resembling a path. I then saw some rustling in the trees and my legs turned to jelly. I was so scared that I ran as fast as I could to the bottom of the mountain.

It began to rain and I was welcomed in by a local family in a mud hut. It was an honour to be invited into their home and I sat next to a small fire while they cooked. I felt privileged to be their guest and to be rescued from the rain.

Later, Luco and I joined a trek in the jungle and were soon in amongst a family of gorillas. A tremendous, crashing and thumping noise was coming towards us from the undergrowth. The Silverback appeared in his majestic way. He took a swipe at the nearest one of our group but was really just giving a warning. We watched the family for a while. It was a joy to see the youngsters frolicking and fooling around, with proud Mum and the great Silverback watching on.

During our time in Rwanda, we were held up at gunpoint. Luco was in charge of our money and I was driving. We were in a sparsely populated area and were suddenly stopped by a gang of armed men. Rwanda was still a dangerous place to be and not long after the genocide. Earlier I had noticed soldiers around and some tanks.

'Hand over our money.' I said to Luco Panicking,

He wouldn't hand over our money and I had little time to think.

'No Joe,' he said, 'take this.'

Instead, he handed me our packed lunch. I then opened the box and offered the bandits a boiled egg through the window. Meanwhile, a small crowd had gathered around and thankfully started to laugh. And that was it! They let us go on our way, saved by a boiled egg.

On our first night in Rwanda, I said to Luco that I appreciated his concern during the Masai incident earlier and he said

' No problem, Joe, Valium takes the edge off things. How about you, do you take anything?'

'I've taken psychiatric pills for years,' I replied.

'Do they have any side effects?'

'Not that I would notice.'

He said, 'I bet my Valium are stronger than your pills.'

'Ok, let's do a swap. 'I said

And so, we did . Luco went quiet for a bit and a bit more. Finally, he said

'Hey Joe,'

'Yes.'

'I can't feel my legs.'

When I think back to that now, I realise I wasn't always so well on that trip and put myself in danger a few times. Through some survival instinct, however, I made my way back to Mary and held on to my sanity just long enough to get back to England.

Chapter 25

The spiritual barterer
direct memories of a mad episode

Did she know I was sent by the holy spirit and guided celestially to her hat and scarf market stall? And did she know that the Messiah had died at the age of thirty-three?

These were the questions in my head. I was in Kingston market.

'How much?' I asked her, as I looked at a colourful hat and scarf. I leant towards her, before she had a chance to answer and whispered, 'Thirty-three.'

I then noticed her move to another section, with different colours. She looked at me for reassurance and with one hand by her side and the other outstretched, she systematically hovered over different sections, like a children's game of 'getting warmer.'

'That's it, 'I said, feeling slightly moved by the whole experience.

She offered the beautiful hat and scarf for forty pounds. I said, 'Thirty-three' and just to trigger the religious significance, I did the sign of the cross and looked at her in a guiding way. She knew, and I knew it would end up being thirty-three pounds and so we exchanged. When I left, she was humming, and I had a skip to my step.

Looking back on this, I can see I wasn't well and I know now from my position of relative sanity that thirty-three pounds was far too much to pay for a hat and scarf. I wonder if she took advantage of me, seeing my odd behaviour. Having others take advantage is a constant danger for those with fragile mental health, as much as any wild encounter in the Serengeti.

Chapter 26

John Trendy and the Folios Foundation

It was the morning of the Barnes village fair. I had little to do, so I decided to go. I wasn't confident and was feeling particularly self-conscious. I just hoped to blend in. I walked straight past a policeman who was laughing and joking with a couple, which helped me relax. Sometimes, little things like that can help.

I trundled on and was beginning to enjoy the fair. So far, so good, I thought. Suddenly, I felt a tight grip on the back of my neck.

'Joe de Souza? 'The voice sounded familiar, but I wasn't sure. I turned around.

'John Trendy!'

We both laughed at the surprise and joy of bumping into each other.

'Joe,' he said, 'you've got to go to the Mind stall over there.' He pointed vaguely.

'Why?' I asked

'My car is parked right behind it and if you guess the weight, you win a prize. You can get three goes for a fiver.'

John Trendy and I went back years. We were altar boys together. More recently, I met him now and again and he would often ask, 'Joe, still on the gear?'

And I would reply. 'Oh yes, it keeps me well.'

He always looked concerned. This went on for a long time until I realised what he meant. Finally, I confronted him.

'John,' I said 'I've never been on hard drugs, if that's what you mean. I continue to take psychiatric medication for my illness.'

He paused, shook his head and said, 'I'll kill my mother.'

I went in the direction of the Mind stall, as John had suggested, but all I could see was a stall for the Samaritans. I chatted to them briefly and they all seemed quite depressed. I asked them where the Mind stall was, and they told me where to go.

At last, I could see it and I could also see John Trendy's car. It was big, more of a truck, and the stall holders showed me a chart with all the suggested weights. I ticked three boxes at random and handed over my fiver.

'Can we have your details?' The woman in charge asked.

I said' No don't worry, if I win, let John Trendy claim the prize.'

So, I walked off and smiled to myself. I was glad that I had contributed to an important charity and one that my friend and I were connected to.

I went home and relaxed. Two hours later, I got a phone call.

' Joe, John Trendy here.'

'Yes.'

'You've won. You guessed the weight of my car.'

'Really?'

'Yeah, I'll be over in a bit with your prize.'

So, half an hour later he was at my place. We had a cuppa, and I eagerly opened the envelope. It read.

The Folios Foundation offers complementary therapies.

Shiatsu

Reflexology

Nutritional advice

Acupuncture

You are entitled to two free sessions.

Dicky Bamford (Founder and Leader)

I decided that it would be a good idea to offer them to my sister Bex and her daughter Ruby. When I did catch up with Bex, she showed some interest, but first decided to check the place out online.

'Joe, it's genuine and it offers therapies to clients with various difficulties, some of whom run the place. I think this is more your cup of tea.'

Finally, I mentioned my dilemma to my great-old friend Jay and he was interested.

'Yeah Joe, I'll come, just let me know when you're booked in and we can go together.'

'By the way Jay, it's in Kings Cross.' I added.

'Cool,' he said.

One afternoon, out of the blue, I got a call.

'Hi Joe, John Trendy here.'

'Oh, Hi, where are you?'

'At the Folios. Yeah man, you've got to get down here. Ooh, me bleeding back... that's better. When are you going to come along?'

'Soon,' I said

Four days later, Jay and I met outside Kings Cross station. I was pleased and relieved to see him.

''Are you sure you don't mind being here?' I asked

'No bother.' he replied

We found the place and it seemed a little inconspicuous. There was no sign above the door and that seemed to make me more nervous. The door was ajar, and I knocked and walked in and immediately spoke to a man behind a desk.

'Hello, my name's Joe de Souza and I won two free health treatments at the Barnes Fair, at the Mind stall, organised by John Trendy.'

There was a moment of utter confusion; I showed the piece of paper, which was signed by their spiritual leader, Dicky Bamford, and it was finally sorted out, despite my surprising entrance. I was indeed booked in. We were early, so we agreed that we'd come back in half an hour.

Jay said that I should have just said 'I've come for my Four thirty appointments.'

I said' It's a bit shady. It's not a brothel, is it?' and he laughed.

I returned on my own, as Jay had now headed back and with trepidation, I entered the building alone.

'Was the receptionist mentally ill? I wondered. I struck up a brief conversation with him and he now knew that my other free ticket was for reflexology. He pointed to a woman standing close by and said 'This is our reflexologist.'

She looked eccentric and her hair was dishevelled and partially covering her eyes. I wondered if she would be able to see my feet clearly. I asked about the shiatsu masseur-

'Is she nearly ready?'

'It's a he.' The man behind the desk replied. Suddenly, a man dressed head to toe in a white gown appeared from almost nowhere, like an apparition. He beckoned me and I followed him into his room. I was relieved to be able to keep my clothes on. Soon, I was lying down and could feel his knees next to my tummy. Nothing was happening, so I barely opened one eye to see what was occurring, hoping he wouldn't notice. He was making strange sweeping body and arm movements as if to clear the air of bad spirits. I wondered if this was a ritual, or perhaps it was to clear the air of body odour. Nonetheless, I tried to remain calm despite being in this weird place and winning my odd prize. I was now really hoping to be back home, or even in a local pub with a nice pint of Guinness. I was probably the most stressed-out client the white-robed masseur had ever encountered.

I finally left the building and as I was walking towards Kings Cross station, I asked myself, why do the funniest and strangest things happen to me?

Chapter 27

Dan and I take a Christmas trip

Dan and I were getting excited about our Christmas trip. But best of all, it was going to be our first Christmas time together in Cornwall. My sister Bex has a house there and it is lovely.

The preparations started a few days earlier, as Dan's Mum, my ex-partner, Michelle, had taken Dan clothes shopping, as he had recently had a growth spurt.

So, kitted out perfectly, Christmas presents in the boot, luggage in the back seat and Santa's sock hidden carefully, we were on our way at about eight am. On other trips we had left much earlier, but my sister Bex had insisted.

'No, you are not leaving at six, the last time you did that, you nearly fell asleep and when you arrived, you fell out of the car sideways like a crab.'

The A303 was no problem. I loved it and was even excited about our average Miles per gallon, the distance covered and in what time.

'We're halfway there and it's only half Ten.' I said

'Really?' Dan replied.

'Yes, and you'll be pleased to hear we've been averaging 50MPG.'

Dan remained silent, apart from the occasional rumbling from his tum. We pulled over to the next service station and Dan had a sandwich and I had a fag and a coffee. We headed on and decided to have one more break before Cornwall and in the meantime, Dan had pulled his jacket over his head and dozed off. The fields were as pretty as a picture and covered in a blanket of snow. Dan continued to snooze, so I didn't stop again, but woke Dan up a little before Boscastle, our destination.

Finally, after five hours, we arrived. We turned one last corner and there was our family. My sister Bex and her husband Nick and their two children, Ruby and George. They had gathered to welcome us like a great big warm glove. They were all delighted and relieved and somehow, I managed to tell them about the trip as if it was an epic adventure, as bold and daring as going to the moon... Dan smiled and Bex had prepared a lovely lunch.

Dan was only six, nearly seven and still believed in Santa and so did his cousin Ruby. When I had a moment, I called them over for a walk to the harbour, which was only a stone's throw from the cottage. I explained to them the method Santa would use to deliver his presents all around the coast.

'It's a very fast but quiet hovercraft so that he can get in and out of the bays silently. If he is ahead of time and he has been spotted doing this only once, he will jump out of his hovercraft and if the waves are right, he will surf them on his sleigh.'

Ruby and Dan were thrilled.

'The Boscastle lighthouse keeper saw this happen one Christmas Eve, when the moon was particularly bright, and the stars shone like sapphires. I think he deserves a little break after all his hard work. Don't you?'

' Yes, but what about his reindeer?' Dan replied.

'The hovercraft is very big and follows him almost magnetically and they're tucked up in bed, below, ready for the huge land journeys. It's been said by the lighthouse keeper that all manner of creatures join in to surf the waves.

' Like what Dad?'

'Oh, porpoises, seals, dolphins and even mermaids'

'Not mermaids. No one believes in them, 'said Ruby

'But when the light catches a porpoise just right-legend says that they swim around shipwrecks, becoming just like mermaids and keep old sailors' company, and rumour has it, that Santa dives deep below the ocean waves and brings little gifts of food to all the sea creatures that are keeping the old sailor's company in their watery graves. Let's go back now.' I said

We arrived back at the house and Nick and George were playing table tennis in the garden. Later, when it began to cool, the fire was lit. They all sat around the fire laughing and joking. Bex was being funny and showing off. I stared at the fire and thought about what I had said to the children. The fire sent out flickers of warmth and it fizzed and popped like a shooting star. Just for a moment, I was alone, on a beach by a fire, overlooking the sunset and was totally at peace.

'Joe, it's ok, they're upstairs and fast asleep. We can do Santa.'

Bex and I snuck upstairs and carefully placed the Santa socks. George was a few years older and he was enjoying the tradition, whilst watching from his room. In half an hour, everybody was asleep.

The next morning, Dan leaped onto my bed 'Dad, look what Santa brought me.'

I woke up quickly and was delighted. I felt proud and happy.

'Do you think he left any footprints?' I asked, but he was already engrossed in Santa presents.

When Dan wasn't looking (or Bex and Nick) I went into the kitchen, picked up a cup, filled it with water and sprinkled it just outside the front door and a little inside.

'Look Dan, he's come up from the harbour.'

Dan was now ecstatic and ran upstairs to get Ruby. After breakfast, they all gathered in the main room and began to open presents to each other. However, Dan had noticed that some of his presents from Santa were in the same wrapping paper as the ones from me. He looked concerned and asked me why that was .'Santa must have been in a terrible rush and borrowed some of my leftover wrapping paper to finish off with.'

Dan seemed mystified and wasn't convinced. Gradually, bit by bit and even on the car journey home, he began the growing-up process of not believing in Father Christmas. At first, he was angry with me, but as soon as he was home, the big hug from his Mum made it all better.

When I think about that Christmas, I feel proud that I was a good Dad to Dan and am grateful to my sister and her family for welcoming us in like that and enabling me to be an even better Dad.

Chapter 28

The respect marshal

Anyone who suffers from mental health issues knows that a few pills can be the difference between being well and extremely unwell. Part of becoming well is about learning to look after yourself. I think I really started to look after myself after the birth of my son Dan. Being a Dad has made me pay attention to my mental health, for his sake.

When he was about ten years old, Dan joined a local football team and was keen to do well. He practised regularly and he really looked forward to match days. There were only really two jobs that the parents had to do: get their kids to the away matches and be responsible for the linesman flags. I was cautious about volunteering but wanted to do my bit, so after a game, I talked to Dan about the flags and asked him whether I should volunteer.

'No,' he said. 'You'll get it completely wrong and you'll be embarrassing, and I really don't want you to.'

I respected his wishes, but it meant that I had to turn up a couple of minutes after the start of the game, to avoid being asked to take care of the flags and risk getting it wrong and embarrassing my son.

One Sunday, Dan's team manager approached me and asked if I would put on the 'Respect Marshall shirt.' It was bright green - fluorescent.

'Certainly,' I said, although I hadn't a clue what it was for. I thought maybe someone had just died.

I agreed to wear it and was told that the job was to monitor any bad behaviour on or off the pitch. I wasn't in the slightest bit nervous; it gave me a sense of purpose and made me feel like I was contributing. Even Dan didn't mind.

The next game, I agreed to wear the shirt in the second half. We were playing a tough team from Feltham and at half-time, I decided to nip to the loo and be back in time for the second half. However, I got locked in the changing rooms by the groundsman.

Not only was there nobody to hear my calls, but I was beginning to feel panicky. I felt trapped. I wondered who I could call. If I called the fire brigade, it would probably stop the match. But if I didn't call anybody, God only knew when I would get out. I had spent many months locked up in hospitals and now I was locked up in the changing rooms at my son's football match. I decided to try and break the lock by barging the door and kicking it. I must have made sufficient noise, as eventually the groundsman rescued me. I was too relieved to be cross.

At half term, Dan went to stay with my sister and I travelled to Ireland to see my great friend Mary. Even though we'd kept in touch; I hadn't seen her for over twenty years and I was emotional about seeing her again as well as very nervous about the flight and the airport procedures. Anyone with anxiety knows that travelling can be stressful. You are not in control and there are a thousand things to worry about. The trip went well and I had a lovely time, however, I'd forgotten to bring my medication with me.

When I returned a few days later, I felt all right and was really looking forward to watching Dan play and to getting back to marshalling with my Respect Marshall Shirt.

However, the combination of missing a few days' worth of pills, the stress of travelling and the big emotional experience of catching up with my old friend had affected me more than I'd realised. As soon as I put on the fluorescent shirt, I felt strangely powerful and was a bit high.

I'm bound to get respect wearing this special shirt, I thought, although that wasn't the point of wearing it. I knew I was a bit off-kilter. So, I focussed on Dan and was able to recover. Getting back and the pills also helped. It was a reminder of the nature of my illness and the pitfalls, but also, my luck.

Chapter 29

Three go mad in Hounslow

I was feeling a bit sensitive. Surely a local shopping trip wouldn't trigger a manic episode.

Pippa, my girlfriend at the time, her son, Ted, and I parked up and walked into the town. We were in a hurry, as we had only an hour and a half on the car meter.

'You go off to the shops,' I said to them

'And I'll meet you outside Mc Donald's in twenty minutes or so. I'll be in the seating area outside.'

I ordered my happy meal and didn't wait long before collection. It was in a boxed container and I took it outside with my coffee so I could smoke afterwards and wait for Pippa and Ted. After I sat down, I was almost immediately joined by a homeless man who placed his sleeping bag on the table next to mine. Then his friend came and then another. The first man looked at me and smiled so broadly he was almost laughing and I didn't know why. Perhaps it was my bright red jacket or the fact that my burger and chips were contained in a box shaped like a castle with a fluffy toy on the side. I decided to move inside.

I finished my food and noticed that the three wise men had disappeared. So, I took my coffee outside and rolled a ciggy. A policeman had appeared at the opposite side of the street, outside the pound shop and an old feeling of paranoia began to set in.

'He can't arrest me for wearing an offensive red jacket', I mused.

Then, two McDonald's managers came out and were looking official and business-like. They stood on either side of me and began to measure the fencing, bordering the seating area adjacent to me.

'Now what's happening?' I thought. 'Surely they're not sizing me up for a coffin? All I've done is go for a burger. Where are Pippa and Ted'

The policeman had disappeared into the pound shop. I was trying to hold onto reality and drink my coffee. Before my coffee was satisfyingly guzzled, Pippa and Ted reappeared. I retold my story to Pippa, and she laughed and said: 'It could only happen to you.'

I smiled with relief. I was back with my friends and walking away from my mad twenty minutes.

We moved further down the high street and Pippa and her son had been distracted, so I took the opportunity to investigate a religious stall, marshalled by an Indian-looking lady. I couldn't resist and soon enough, she couldn't resist praying for me either. But first, she seemed to want something to pray for and I told her a little bit about myself. Although she seemed a bit bemused, we were very soon holding hands and praying together.

Pippa and Ted were only up the road and they could see me holding hands and praying with a complete stranger and I had only been gone two minutes.

After my brief meeting with the religious lady, Pippa said she wanted to get her eyebrows done. So, Ted and I agreed to wait nearby to while away the time. Fifteen minutes later, Pippa reappeared, and her eyebrows looked fine.

Now was the time for them to get some shopping done at the Supermarket, so they went on to shop. I needed a lighter, so I went into a convenience store, close by and went up to the manager who was serving.

'Yes,' he said

'Oh yes, I'd like a lighter.' He peered behind him.

'Yes,' I said. 'That one with the cannabis leaves on it would be fine.'

His assistant giggled.

'One pound please,' he said, but he didn't look pleased.

I offered him a pound, but it was from the old currency.

'No,' he said crossly, and I realised my mistake.

'Ooh I'm terribly sorry' I gave him the correct money and left. However, the manager followed me out and, just as I was leaving, I paused to look at the window display and heard him shouting:

'You bring confusion to my shop. Get out!'

I turned to see what was going on, but it was me he was shouting at.

Pippa and Ted soon reappeared, and, when I had explained what had happened, Pippa said,

'We've all been there.'

I don't know if that's true. Not everyone has been there. Pippa and her son suffer from mental health difficulties, that's why she was able to reassure me. It is one of the problems we face when we go out in public. Other people treat us either with disrespect or react the way that manager did, with aggression. Most of the time, we are simply trying to get by and do a bit of shopping.

Chapter 30

The Cornish sea and the seagull

I regularly go to Cornwall, where my sister has a house. I remember one trip to Trebarwith, a local beach.

I dived into the cold refreshing sea and felt the bubbling froth left behind by the last wave, stirred up like a witch's cauldron. I was up to my waist.

'Do the waves get bigger when the tide goes out?' I remember my son Dan asking me before he got in. He was frolicking in the shallow surf with his cousin Ruby and I didn't really know.

I dived under a wave. That was the best bit. Just as good as catching and riding one, as elegantly as the sea would allow. I looked back and could still see them playing around in the shallows close to the shore. They were perhaps fifty yards away now.

I had learnt to be aware of the depth I was in and would often quickly retreat far enough back for my feet to touch the ocean floor.

A big wave broke over me and now I was clearly out of my depth with the swell that followed. I was nervous, especially as I was without flippers, which would always help my body surfing, confidence and buoyancy. This time though, I didn't have that aid and I had barely been able to recover from the first wave when another came thundering down on top of me. I fought all instincts not to panic. I was being tossed around like a ragdoll in a tumble drier.

'Fuck elegance, 'I thought. ' I just want to breathe.'

And then the next one. They seemed to be getting bigger and I could feel the surf pulling me out to sea. The tide was on the turn and Dan and Ruby were out of sight. I was thrashing and suffocating and praying for dear life.

The sea began to calm. The sun seemed to shine just a little brighter and by some miracle the final wave picked me up and seemed to place me onto a sandbank as if to save my life. It was like an oasis in a vast watery desert. So far removed from that terrible tide. I could feel soft sand beneath my toes. I was standing in mere inches of water, which would fill and drain with each passing movement of the sea.

A lone seagull appeared from a distance and hovered directly above me. I looked up and watched it dip and skip in the sky, but it was neither flying forward nor back. It stayed the same, in the same spot. It followed me from high, even as I walked back to shore. Then I saw Dan and Ruby and waved. They returned my wave and continued playing happily.

When I finally reached the beach, the seagull squawked and flew high into the sky and took a sharp turn back towards a dusky setting sun. It flew away effortlessly and beautifully, on a current of air, until it became a mere speck on the horizon and then it was gone.

Chapter 31
Glad you're still with us
(around 1983)

It only seemed a breath away, that I was sitting on the back of my brother's moped and flying down the tunnel at Hyde Park. We were on our way back from a shift at Mc Donald's in the Haymarket. We were doing sixty miles an hour and I was fifteen years old. I clung tight to Tim and closed my eyes. I could feel every movement: the tilt of the bike, the bumps in the road and the cool wind in my face .

I met my first girlfriend Maggie at McDonald's and enjoyed the camaraderie of working with not just my brother but several new faces as well. I learnt about the value of money and managed to save up a hundred pounds towards a family skiing holiday.

But now, three and a bit years later, I was in a psychiatric hospital and was missing my family and friends. After a few months in an acute lock up ward, my mental health had improved, and I had been transferred back to an open ward and was allowed out. I decided to ask the staff for some leave for a few hours, so that I could play golf.

'Yes, Joe, but make sure to be back on time.'

I took out a small bag of clubs that my Dad had brought in for me previously. I was excited and although I had a huge sticker with my name emblazoned onto my bag, there wasn't anything all that different about me, except my mind. I was normally good with golf etiquette. However, I was on a new course and in my state anything could happen. I queued up to play and was confronted by a man who was probably an official of the club.

'Where are your shoes?"

'Here.' I gestured towards my trainers.

'You can't play in them.'

I panicked, jumped in front of the queue and legged it across the golf course.

'Oi!' I heard him shout. 'Come back here. What are you on?'

Presumably many of the other golfers watched this young man being chased across their golf course, like a spooked, fleeing rabbit.

It isn't the only time, when pursuing one of my hobbies, that misunderstanding has ensued. As well as golf, I have always loved fishing. In fact, I recently tried to renew my membership with a fishing club in Surrey.

'Hello,' the man's voice echoed loudly down the line.

'Oh yes,' I said. 'Hello. Is that the club secretary?'

'Yes, it is indeed.'

'Oh good,' I said, 'I'm hoping to renew my membership again this year. My name is Joe de Souza.'

'Fantastic, John. Do you have an OAP concession?'

I wondered why he was calling me John and why he assumed I was an OAP.

'No, but I do have a concession for a disability. (I tried to tone it down a bit) Anxiety and depression.'

He said, 'We've got a couple of cracking specialist disability swims at one of our bigger waters.'

A swim is the name of the area on the bank from where you are going to fish from and the area in front of you in the water that you wanted to fish. Now I was almost giggling. I had no idea what a specialist disability swim could possibly entail. How can a fishing lake accommodate a psychiatric condition? Do they have a voice box next to the swim and every hour a calming subliminal message comes out of the system?

'Don't worry you will catch a fish! '

Or perhaps a box of pills appeared from a little hole in the riverbank with a written message like Alice in Wonderland: please, take me. '

Needless to say, I joined. Partly because the club secretary was so funny. I realise now he must have meant an access ramp or something, but I remember the last thing he said was:

'Glad to hear you're still with us.'

Chapter 32

Love, Dan and redemption

I was always a natural show off and an extravert. If a nervous breakdown would arise, it would often show my personality in an exaggerated form. Extravagant and extreme forms of behaviour for example. Some people would retreat into themselves and some may become overly aggressive. Anxiety and depression are two severe symptoms of illness that would often go hand in hand. They can both reflect an inability to express anger and this bottled-up anger would be turned inwards. Psychosis is a more severe form of this. When the brain is overloaded with stress and at crisis point, it protects itself and reverts to a coping mechanism, which can become mental illness. Our ego becomes fractured; the subconscious takes over to compensate. Our mind sees reality in a distorted, dreamlike or nightmarish way. It's confusing, dangerous and frightening.

During my breakdowns, along with many other symptoms, I became grandiose. In other words, I had delusions of grandeur. When I was very young, and suffering my first big breakdown, I was convinced I was Jesus. That delusion returned repeatedly, possibly due to my religious upbringing. I felt God was communicating to me through the TV and giving me signs. For example, John McEnroe shouted at the umpire during Wimbledon was joining and shouting with me – he was sharing this with me. I also read signs in day-to-day life that it could be someone putting on their shoes or making a cup of tea, and to me, that was a sign from God. My subconscious took over my reality. Once, I flooded the bathroom by doing a running dive into the bath, to test my faith and courage. I would shout at anyone who disagreed with me, including visitors. I'd show a friend or family member a poem that I had recently written, and when their reaction wasn't to my liking, I'd be furious.

'That's a work of art, 'I would say. 'How dare you.'

But Jesus was loving, patient and forgiving. Not mad, impatient and rude. I became less and less like Jesus. In the middle of my crisis, I became frustrated at being locked up and without knowing anything about the pills I was taking, became heavily drugged. One of the new drugs that I had been given was called Largactil. It was referred to by the patients as the Liquid Cosh. My limbs became achy and heavy and I felt fatigued. My speech was affected and I began to slur my words. Although by now, I was allowed out of the ward to visit the social centre, even though I could barely walk. I began to feel so exhausted that I fell in a crumpled heap on the floor in the middle of an empty courtyard. A good Samaritan came to my aid. It was a woman who was working nearby and she helped me back on my feet and to the centre.

Eventually, my grandiose fantasy began to subside. I woke up in the dorm one morning and asked myself,

'Am I Jesus Christ or Joe de Souza?'

I decided I was Joe de Souza. From that moment, my mental health began to improve. It was a relief to be me again, but also mildly painful. Reality sucked. Now I was just stuck in the hospital, the same as everyone else.

As I began to recover, it was a great relief to go home for a night or two. One time, it was during the festive season. My sister Bex and I always put up a Christmas list of fake requests, which always made us laugh. Roller skates for Dad and poster paints for Mum for example. It was always good to see my family and I loved them.

By the end of my psychiatric journey, I had been hospitalised ten or so times, including being sectioned, for six months, four times. I spent nearly three years in hospital and had about a dozen breakdowns.

And then in 2002 my son was born and my new life emerged like a butterfly from a cocoon. His birth broke the cycle of hospital stays and periodic breakdowns and now, years later, we can enjoy the warmth and laughter of family together. On one occasion recently, Mum had invited Dan and I for supper.

'Great,' I said. ' We'll be over just after five.'

Both Mum and I are punctual. I picked up Dan just before five by car and we set off. We chatted together and managed to find a parking space just outside their house.

Whenever we went around there, Dad would always be sitting in his usual chair in the kitchen, at the bottom of some steps, descending from the garden. I would always cough or call his name, as I'd walk towards him, so as not to give him a fright. They are both in their eighties.

Dan finds them both sweet and funny and we both look forward to seeing them.

I coughed and Dad slid out of his chair to open the door and sat back down. There was no time for greetings as he immediately announced,

'I am very upset about the tomatoes.'

'Why?' we asked

'I've been made to peel a lot of tomatoes and I prefer the canned ones. I like the flavour of the tin.'

Mum interrupted: 'Hello darlings, I've cooked a delicious meal and we've even got fresh tomatoes. How are you both?'

Dan and I looked at each other and smiled.

'That sounds great. Yeah, we're both fine.'

I laughed inwardly and sensed this was going to be a battle of the tomatoes, which I knew Mum would win. As we sat down for supper, I could see that Mum was pleased with what she had produced, but as soon as she sat down, she accused Dad of not liking the tomatoes because he had to peel them. Nobody spoke and then she said

'It's rather nice, isn't it, Teddy?'

And Dad replied, 'Absolutely delicious darling.'

'Yes, especially with the fresh tomatoes,' she added

A very short time later she said, 'I think this is restaurant standard.'

Dan and I remained quiet, especially as we knew that the spaghetti was slightly overcooked.

We enjoyed the meal and then I realised there was pudding. I served all four of us and we tucked in. Although it was shop bought, it was delicious; a simple chocolate tart with custard, I barely looked up to speak. Plus, I was making appreciative murmurs due to its deliciousness. Mum interrupted my bliss. She leant over the table towards me and said

'Are you glad you came over *now*?'

I think she was annoyed that I preferred the shop-bought pudding to her main meal. At this point, both me and Dan began to laugh, and Mum seemed rather surprised.

Chapter 33

In and out of madness 1980 - 2000

Mum's role in my countless recoveries was huge. She refused to feel sorry for me and continued her tough love stance. If I escaped from the hospital in Epsom and made my way home to Barnes, she would unhesitatingly turn me away and send me back.

'You're not supposed to be here,' she would say. ``Go back to hospital and I'm not going to give you a lift.'

There was a time when I arrived on their doorstep and unbeknownst to me, the police were called.

'I belong here,' I said, disappointed and upset. 'In my home, not locked up. What is happening?'

The more I shouted, the less I was listened to. It was an ongoing occurrence. Mum or Dad would try and explain.

'Joe, you have to go back. You are unwell and when you're well and ready, you can come home.'

I spoke to Mum recently who told me it was very upsetting and shocking – police, ambulances, neighbours, plus the sight of her son so distressed and confused. But it was completely fair, as I was on a section, which meant I had been taken into hospital for my own safety, and the rules had to apply. Perhaps out of sensitivity to my parents or the fact that I was ill rather than a criminal, the police would let me out of my parents' front door so that I could walk calmly towards the police wagon at the bottom of the paved path. But I remember one time, just as I reached them, the fight or flight reaction possessed me and I tried to flee. But no sooner had I made a break for it than I was picked up like a feather and placed in the back of the wagon, to be driven back to the hospital in Epsom.

I remember feeling no fear on that occasion. In fact, I felt quite calm and strangely important – the sirens were on and there were three big policemen in the van with me. I suppose I had my own police escort! I still didn't really understand but the police and the sirens accompanying me, were also a big reminder that I needed to become well to get my freedom back.

After leaving her job as a presenter on children's TV, Mum changed careers and moved to the Citizens Advice Bureau. She often helped me with forms that I couldn't decipher; partly because I was too poorly to read... One form was unintelligible, and ridiculously complex. I was nineteen at the time and Mum took a stand and went as far as getting a letter published in the Guardian. Suspiciously soon, I was granted the correct amount of money with no further ado.

Dad was still behaving like a funny and eccentric film star . Years earlier, I remember being in the school playground and seeing him at the gates. He had come to pick me up in his seventies style bathing trunks and nothing else. I was too young to be embarrassed, in fact I felt very proud. He walked towards me as easily as a city office worker would walk to work in a pinstripe suit.

For a long while, mental illness was a thing that I became used to. It had become my life. If I wasn't hanging around with friends that I had met in hospital, I would be visiting friends inside the hospitals that I had known from previous admissions.

An episode would tend to often occur when I was either bored or vulnerable. On these occasions, I was more comfortable in the hospital surroundings, especially if I wasn't myself. Clearly, for me, there was wellness on the outside, illness on the inside, and a big grey area in between. I would spend so much time visiting the mentally ill that soon enough, I would be admitted myself. Mental illness can be catching, in that sense. The visitor can become the visited. I know that happened to me.

It makes me think of the book 'Catch 22', which rang true, the idea that you must be mad to want to be in an asylum.

Many times, my behaviour would partly be a cry for help. An instinct for survival and self-preservation would kick in. Hospitals can be dangerous, there is the risk of being attacked by others, especially young men, who are very ill - but I felt safe there.

The submission ward was less severe than the lock-up ward. The more ill you became, the more likely it was you would be sent to the more acute, but sometimes safer, environment. The more acute wards were safer because of the specialist nursing care.

On any ward and at any time, I could communicate with very ill patients. It was as if we had a secret language, which I couldn't comprehend when I was well and which outsiders couldn't understand. There was a kindred spirit between the patients. Words and phrases were bandied around like 'sixth sense' or 'magic'. to describe certain people – and we all knew what we meant.

I may have understood a lot about the vulnerable, but I didn't always make good judgments. My new friendships weren't always appropriate but because of my blinkered state, I couldn't tell.

What would come to me in time, was that I too was locked up and my choices of friends inside were not always ideal on the outside. That was a hard thing to come to terms with.

Life continued and I would get to hear snippets of news from my siblings. Dad would maybe be starring in a new play, or film, or radio. He was at his best when acting when he remembered to go to work. I can remember one of my siblings telling me that Dad had almost missed a gig - one Saturday, he'd been relaxing in the kitchen with a roll up and a coffee when Mum had burst into the room and cried:

'Teddy, what are you doing?'

'I'm having a cup of coffee.'

'But you've got to go to work, you're at the National Theatre.'

'But not until later.'

'It's a matinee!'

'Oh Crikey.'

During the periods between sections and hospital stays, I would often attend day centres. I went off and on for several years. There would be a gathering of regulars, a basic lunch and cheap teas. It was a way of life for many. It was a community. Stepping outside of that community meant entering into society where people had less understanding of mental illness and vulnerability. I would sometimes take people out of those safe groups and into the wider world for a day trip, which was exciting for them. During my thirties, my flat would often be full of people from this community – I was not quite as ill as many of them and could help them, in a way. I felt popular and it was fun, but it wasn't necessarily good for me in terms of my health.

About this time, there was a gathering of some of Mum's relatives, which was becoming rarer because of the natural ageing process. It was a posh crowd and I could hear a lot of *oh jolly goods*. And a variety of expressions that sounded like an old fifties war movie – not quite *we're going to hit Gerry and we're going to hit him hard* - but that type of thing.

One of the relatives had cornered Mum and asked a direct question.

'How are your children doing?'

'Oh marvellously, thank you. Tim's won all sorts of awards for his Business in Australia and has a wonderful house and wife, plus two lovely children. Lu is incredibly successful as a GP and practically runs the NHS. Bex is doing exceedingly well as chief executive of Tiger Aspect.'

'What about Joe?'

'He's a champion day centre attender and has reduced his days from four to three.'

The woman looked slightly crestfallen, but Mum was as proud as punch.

Chapter 34
Daniel

Daniel's Mum and I lived in the same block and were next-door neighbours. We had a brief fling which resulted in her getting pregnant and we broke up shortly afterwards. At the time, I wasn't ready for fatherhood, and I had become ill – this is going back nineteen years. Because of my poor mental health, my ex was uncomfortable about me seeing Daniel on my own so I could only see him with her there or one of my sisters or my mother. I can't remember too much of the detail, but I must have known deep down that this was for the best.

When he did arrive, I remember vividly holding him and feeling that my life was beginning to turn around. I felt a purpose. This is my son, I thought. It didn't happen overnight but the more I held him in my arms, the more I changed. Because of him, within a short time, I grew up. Gone was the reckless behaviour, now I looked forward to seeing him and the best way to see him was to behave responsibly – and that meant looking after myself. A big step was to recognise that alcohol didn't agree with me or my meds. I stopped drinking. I stopped hanging around with my ill friends, took the meds regularly and made myself available at a moment's notice – all huge changes but I made them because of Daniel, because I wanted to be part of his life.

I kept up my decision to look after myself and began to enjoy better mental health as a result. In time, I was allowed to take Daniel out in the car and together with his mother, we would sometimes go and see my sister Lu in Watford. She would teach Daniel how to bake a cake and I always felt proud of him. On the way back to London, I would pass a few slices over to his Mum and Daniel would often suggest that he look after the cake in the backseat - for safe keeping on the way home!

We were bonding with each visit. Eventually, I can't remember exactly how old he was – maybe about three or four – I was able to be with him on my own. His mother would leave him at my flat and we would practise golf putting or throwing balls into a target. His favourite thing to do was stand on the bed while I ran across the room and did a dramatic commando roll . In fact, it was just head-over-heels and then I waited for him to jump on me, which he thought was hilarious.

My sister Bex fussed over him just as much as Lu, and Daniel got on well with her daughter Ruby. I remember taking him over to Bex's after one of his first days at big school. He was five and he did look adorable. But I think the school tie sealed it. She opened the door and nearly melted.

Soon, we were invited on holiday to Bex's place in Cornwall and I was allowed to drive both Dan and I to their home in Boscastle. I found the journey there with Dan just as fun and bonding as the holiday itself as I savoured these moments with him.

Often, we would go to our local pool. At one point a staff member asked where he was born, and he said, 'Australia', which tickled me. (Years later, I did take him to Australia to visit my brother Tim and relatives.) But as we were leaving the swimming pool, they called out.

'See you.'

And Dan replied, 'Love you.'

He was about four. As he got older, we went fishing together and I couldn't have been happier, although we didn't completely agree on who caught the *biggen*. But somehow, he did prevent me from falling in.

More recently we went camping together and spent time chatting together before our makeshift fire at night and swimming in the clear Dorset Sea during the day.

One of my favourite trips with Daniel was to Brighton. When we arrived on the beach, there was no time for sunbathing, especially as the funniest thing in the world for Dan was to tip a load of pebbles down the back of my shirt. I would exaggerate my reaction of shock horror, which delighted him. That's also where he first learnt to swim. He was about four at the time. I was in the sea up to my waist, and I called to him, come on, swim to me. And he launched himself towards me and – I think maybe due to blind trust - just swam. It was like a miracle, and one of the loveliest moments I've ever had.

> Today, writing these memories, I realise that these are perfectly normal memories of a Dad and his boy, it's simply that I know how hard-won they were.

Daniel gave me my life back. My life had been missing, in a way, for twenty-two years. My life really did begin at forty.

Recently, he was accepted at University, and I am always happy to pick him up from or drive him to Bristol. This is another big stage in his life. His Mum and I are still friends and fortunately for all of us, he has love from both sides of the family.

He does understand that I've got an illness, and he knows that I've written about it, although I haven't told him everything. I think he sees it as more of an exaggerated eccentricity, like his actor grandpa and how the humour brings us closer. But he often talks to me as a friend, as well as a son and I feel love and respect towards him as much as any parent would.

In the last Father's Day card that I received; he had written.

'Thank you, Dad, for always being there for me .' It was heartfelt and honest, and I was moved by it.

And it's true, I will always be there for him.

Conclusion

One of the first hurdles that I encountered when I became ill, was accepting that I was ill. Especially as I was deluded and thought I was perfectly well. It became very difficult for friends and family members to persuade me otherwise. It was better for all concerned, to nip it in the bud. Unfortunately for me, the build-ups and the sleepless nights were a path to destruction. I finally succumbed to my illness and would be hospitalised.

Mental illness can range from eating disorders to addictions and various degrees of anxiety and depression, OCD, delusions and psychosis... There is often a cross over when an illness covers different headings or labels. That is particularly difficult for the doctors and then treating the patient it is often a case of trial and error. At first, I was treated for schizophrenia, then manic depression (bipolar) and then a combination of the two.

Mental health care has improved dramatically in the last forty years and the old-fashioned asylums that I was once in have been replaced by more modern hospitals that are far more patient-friendly. I recently heard that you even have a shower in your own room.

Initially, no one in my family had any experience or understanding of this diabolical illness. So, when I was allowed out for times with them, it was a big relief for me but a big test for them.

After a short weekend at home, my Mum came for a consultation with the hospital staff to see how things had gone. The doctors wanted to know how I had been.

The top psychiatrist opened the meeting...

'Hello, Mrs de Souza. How was Joe over the weekend?'

'Completely bloody bananas,' was her reply.

That sounds old fashioned now but it's helpful to look mental illness in the eye and not be afraid of it. Thank goodness society is opening its eyes to these fairly common and difficult illnesses. It's not over when you're discharged from the hospital, as it can then be a slow recovery process; a stumbling block of small steps on the journey back, and if you're lucky, to a resemblance of your old self.

I hope my collection of short stories goes somewhere towards opening people's minds to the various conditions and the unusual journey that some people have to travel just to be well. Although It's not all doom and gloom and hopefully, this contrast between despair and hope, can be seen through a reflection of some of my experiences and those of my vulnerable friends too.

For anyone struggling with mental health difficulties; you're not alone. It's much more acceptable and less stigmatised. Like life, there are ups and downs and there is light, laughter and love, during and after mental illness.

Epilogue

I enjoyed writing 'No Ordinary Joe 'and had no painful flashbacks. I wrote each chapter in bite-sized chunks.

The pattern of the beginning of each breakdown was like a choreographed film. Everyone close to me played their part and had their say, but no one could really stop it, or know what the outcome would be. I was like an express runaway train, building momentum, but with no emergency stop. Except for the locked doors of a psychiatric hospital.

When my son was born, it changed everything. Gone was my reckless behaviour. I calmed down and even began to take the meds regularly, particularly the Lithium and the injections.

Being a Dad has rescued me from a path of illness and given me my life back.

About the Author

Jonathan Job de Souza (people call him Joe) had a varied and colourful history, including many years spent in and out of hospital suffering from bi-polar disorder. However, his life turned around with the birth of his son and he hasn't been in hospital since. He calls himself semi-retired from being a sports teacher, youth worker and even an ambulance driver for a day centre.